# The Healing Sound of Music

## Kate & Richard Mucci

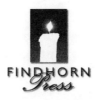

FINDHORN
*Press*

First published by Findhorn Press in 2000

ISBN 1-899171-33-9

British Library Cataloguing-in-Publication Data.
A catalogue record for this book is available from the British Library.

Library of Contress Catalog Card Number: 00-105099


Layout by Pam Bochel
Cover design by Thierry Bogliolo
Front cover painting "En Résonnance" by Jac Lapointe


Printed and bound by Rose Printing, Tallahassee, Florida


Published by
**Findhorn Press**

The Park, Findhorn                    P.O. Box 13939
Forres IV36 3TY                          Tallahassee
Scotland                        Florida 32317-3939, USA
Tel 01309 690582                    Tel 850 893 2920
Fax 01309 690036                    Fax 850 893 3442
e-mail info@findhornpress.com
**findhornpress.com**

# Table of Contents

# Table of Contents

# TABLE OF CONTENTS

♪ *Inner peace is attained by holding loving thoughts*
*about ourselves and others.*
*If we hold those positive, peaceful thoughts,*
*our physical reality will change and it, too,*
*will become peaceful and whole.* ♪

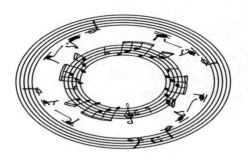

# Preface

How many times have you wondered, "Why am I here?" Why do you think that you chose (or were chosen) to come to this planet at this time? Were you supposed to be a world famous biological researcher, win the Nobel Peace Prize, or fly the first manned mission to the stars? What effect does your existence here on this Earth have in the grand scheme of things? You must have wondered. We don't know many people who haven't taken at least a few moments of their lives to ponder the question.

Usually the answer is an achievement or an accomplishment. Saving the wolves, raising a family, building an international corporation. Those are among the reasons we feel we are here. Many people achieve great things; many even feel that they are doing what they're supposed to do while they're here. But a nagging feeling deep inside, a feeling that something is missing, often taints those accomplishments.

Earning a living, raising a family or maybe even trying to save the planet leaves little time for reflection and soul searching. Unchecked, that "something's missing" feeling can fester into a gnawing discontent, an unshakable depression, or even an overpowering urge to run away.

Some people escape with alcohol and drugs. Others travel to far off places, feeling that everything will be better if they can just find that "perfect place" for two weeks a year. But the temporary high of a lusty affair, a designer drug, or a walk along a Jamaican beach are poor substitutes for the sustained high of genuine joy and peace that comes from within.

While it is true that many places we visit may be beautiful and may even give us a sense of peace for awhile, the return to everyday life can be a harsh jolt. The "high" dies quickly. The feeling is gone. Then it takes more drugs, more money, more acquisitions, more exotic locations, perhaps even exotic people to achieve that feeling again. The discontent can become very painful, indeed, leading to depression or any one of a number of physical ailments.

We spent years trying to fill the void between materialistic accomplishments and true happiness. We were always searching for the ultimate purpose, the final achievement, the flashiest car, the most toys. But during that search, we came upon a Great Truth, and it has been, for us, a catharsis.

We have learned that fulfillment of our purpose on Earth is measured not by the degree or number of our accomplishments nor by material possessions. The joy we experience, and that which we bring to others while traveling on our life's path—that is the true measure of our worth. And the greatest way to bring joy to ourselves and others is, to be at peace.

The peace for which we search is found not on a cruise ship, or in shopping malls, not even in the depths of an ancient redwood forest. It is within. And, it is only when our souls are truly at peace that our bodies and minds can experience the perfect health, joy, and wonder that is our birthright.

All the things that this human experience offers is ten, no, a thousand times better when you are healthy and at peace. The beauty of a sunrise, the artistry of a spider's web, the wrinkles on your grandmother's face. They all take on a magnificence you never believed possible.

The journey to inner peace and health is a personal one. No one can take you there, but we can lead you to the door. Go through it with us now, and you will learn to use the most wondrous gift from the universe—MUSIC to heal, to love,and to embark on your own personal journey to health and happiness.

♪ *Music is the harmonious voice of creation;*
*an echo of the invisible world;*
*one note of a divine chord*
*which the entire universe*
*is destined one day to sound.*

*Mazzini* ♪

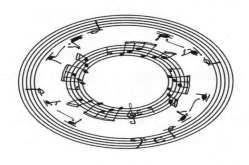

# Introduction

## Hello from Kate

Just recently I was interviewed for an Albuquerque, New Mexico newspaper article, and the reporter asked, "Whatever got you started doing this work? Why the harp?" I was very grateful for his questions, because they made me really think about how we got started in all this.

Ten years ago, I was a typical "yuppie" businesswoman. I owned a service firm doing post-production work for the movie industry. I also had invested in a couple of small businesses that took up much more of my time and energy than I had planned to devote to them.

I was stressed, anxious, and having many physical problems. I worked twelve hours a day, six or seven days a week, and I hardly ever saw Richard. I would sporadically and halfheartedly try to sort out my life by contemplating my own spirituality and the mysteries of life. But I didn't really learn anything, and I stayed caught up in the life I had built. I was always looking for the next contract or trying to pacify an employee who was upset about something.

To be perfectly honest, I was miserable and looking for a way out. But I couldn't see any viable options; I became increasingly unhappy and depressed.

So one night, when I was finally able to get to bed, I lay there crying and praying. I asked God to please help me. I couldn't go on much longer. I knew there must be something else in life. I cried until I finally fell asleep, exhausted, hoping for a miracle.

That night I had a dream. I was playing a harp! I was laughing, relaxed, and happy in that dream. When I awakened, I knew what I had to do.

The next morning, I announced to Richard that I had to get a harp. He very nearly choked on his morning coffee, you can be sure! But being the supportive husband and soul mate that he is, he said we'd find one. And we did.

How can I describe the feeling I got when my little Celtic harp arrived? When I opened the shipping crate, it was the first time I had ever seen a harp up close. I didn't even know how to hold it. But I knew as I touched it, that this was my destiny, and somehow it was going to change my life.

Soon after I began playing, Richard picked up his guitar and played with me. What a beautiful combination it was, and we enjoyed the togetherness of this musical hobby.

Within a year, my physical problems were history. I was smiling again, and we were performing in coffee houses, trendy restaurants, and at festivals and shows. Shortly after our first paying engagement, I sold or closed down all of my businesses, and Richard closed down his radio talent agency. On a wing and a prayer, we left California and went to Las Vegas, Nevada, where Crosswynd took off.

Las Vegas may seem like a strange place to play the kind of music we do, but it was meant to be. After all, is there anywhere else on Earth we could have played for and touched so many people?

As we learned more about spirituality, health, and music, we tried to incorporate what we were learning into our daily work as entertainers. Soon, circumstances and coincidences led us to healing work, and we began practicing healing music and helping people with a myriad of problems.

We didn't really understand how this power of music worked, but we knew that healing was happening because of it. People felt better physically, emotionally, and spiritually, and we were grateful to be a part of their experience.

We were learning what the ancients had known all along...that music was essential to life, health, and happiness. And we felt strongly that we needed to share it with everyone, not just the few we could actually meet and teach in person.

And so, this book is in your hands now. Read it, play the music, learn to use this wondrous power of music to find the peace that will heal your body and soothe your soul.

In Love, and Light, and Peace through Music

Kate Mucci<br>
Santa Fe, New Mexico, September 1999

## Hello from Richard

For years, I thought that music for peace and healing was the latest John Denver song. After all, my world revolved around the music scene as a folk rock guitar player, and a pop music radio announcer.

Shortly after meeting Kate, I found her listening to music that ranged from Handel to Neil Diamond's *"Jonathan Livingston Seagull."*[1] I'd never heard anything like it. It was so comforting.

Later, when Kate began playing the Celtic harp, I heard those same peaceful tones in the music she was learning. I put down my Stratocaster and picked up my acoustic guitar. We began playing this music together and the result was magical. We knew right away that we needed to share it with others.

For the first couple of years, we couldn't put a label on the type of music we were playing and now writing. It wasn't pop, it wasn't Celtic, and it wasn't really new age. This music was about ENERGY! It had to do with tones, vibrations, the feel of music. We began researching and learning more about the power of the kind of music we were playing.

[1] Jonathon Livingston Seagull, CBS, Inc. 1973

I learned that for thousands of years, music, tones, and vibrations were used to heal, transform, and comfort. Music was a huge part of life and health. But somewhere during human evolution, music was pushed aside. It became valued as entertainment only, relegated to parlors and concert halls, removed from the healing process. This wonderful tool to soothe the soul and heal the self fell by the wayside; its magical powers neglected and even forbidden.

Thankfully, not everyone forgot about the healing power of music. In many primitive cultures, it was continually utilized in ceremony, for healing, and for spiritual purposes. In the past several years, we, and musicians like us, re-discovered this secret power of music.

Kate and I see firsthand how men and women are overcome with emotion while listening to our music. We see people become joyful and full of peace. Children sit quietly, comforted by the gentle tones.

A filing cabinet sits in our office. It is full of letters from people in all walks of life, from every corner of the world who have purchased our recordings. They tell us how they've used our music for emotional strength and healing in time of need.

As we read these heartwarming accounts, we realized that this pure, simple, universal music was offering much more than a pleasant listening experience. Our music was helping people. So, we put together much of the information we've gathered after years of research, recording, holding workshops and performing, and presented it to you here, along with a copy of our CD, "*Millennium.*"

Please, use this information and music to heal your body and get in touch with your inner self. Share it with your children and co-workers. Share it with your troubled teenager. Use this book and it's included music like a daily dose of vitamins. It will change your life and help you along a most wonderful journey... to health and the peace within.

Richard J. Mucci
Las Vegas, Nevada, September 1999

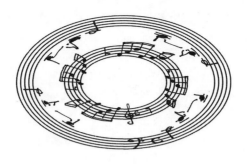

# Space Oddity

Between 1977 and 1989 Voyagers 1 and 2 set out to explore our solar system. What they found was astounding. Although space is a virtual vacuum, and traditional wisdom says that sound cannot exist in a vacuum, Voyager 1 and 2 found plenty of sound.

Sound does indeed exist in space... *as electronic vibrations.*

These sounds are created from solar winds, from the magnetosphere, from trapped radio waves, from charged particle interactions of the planet, its moons, and from charged particle emissions from the rings of certain planets.

NASA released recordings of the sounds that the Voyagers recorded on their five billion mile journey throughout the solar system, creating incredible soundscapes. While they may sound alien or haunting, they are at the same time strangely familiar to the human ear.

In these electronic tones we hear the sounds of human voices singing, winds, waves, birds, and dolphins. Most incredible, one can hear the sound of a harp being played by the celestial wind.

All this from a vacuum?

*Music is God's best gift to man,*
*the only art of Heaven given to earth,*
*the only art of earth that we take to Heaven.*

Charles W. Landon

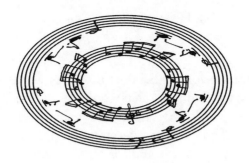

# ONE

# Music Through the Ages

*"Music is the harmony of heaven and earth
and belongs to the higher spiritual realms."*

Yueh Chi

Did you know that the major part of the Chinese character for medicine is the same as the character for music? And the characters representing music and happiness are exactly the same? This connection makes a great deal of sense, if you understand the reverence ancient civilizations had for music and for those who created it.

For these people, music was considered essential for survival. Musicians were shamans, physicians, healers, and priests. They were indispensable. The musician/shaman was respected and revered. In return, they took the spiritual and physical well-being of their charges very seriously. They considered their healing work a spiritual practice. Music and morality were inextricably connected, and they knew that their intentions with the music and their attitude toward those they were healing, was just as important as the music they played and the ceremonies they performed.

The ancients knew that music and sound had great power over the spirit world, the natural world including the plants and animals, and human life. Music was regarded as the force that could bring about harmony in the mind and body of man. Harmony within the community of man—even in the heavenly bodies themselves—was dependent upon music.

The myths of all civilizations say that music came from God, or the heavens. Never is it said to have originated from humans. Sound, especially music that was heard here on Earth, was just a reflection of something taking place beyond the world they knew and understood—some kind of vibratory energy that was the foundation for all that existed.

*"Music, the greatest gift
that mortals know,
And all of heaven
we have below."*

Joseph Addison

Because music could induce trance states, heal, restore harmony, and purify the soul, civilizations from aboriginal Australia to ancient Greece had great myths and legends explaining its power and purpose.

Many ancient peoples believed that sound created the universe. The Hopis believed that it was a song that created the world; the Australian aborigines believed that the Creator beat upon the seas with a reed and thereby created the universe. In Indian mythology, the whole universe "hangs on sound." For them, sound creates letters, words, language, and therefore human life.

Greek mythology is full of references to the awesome power of music. Apollo was the God of the Sun, but he was also the founder of medicine and music. He invented the lyre, and his son, Orpheus, was the first to learn to play it. Orpheus was responsible for calming the beasts of the underworld with his music. Aeseulapius, Apollo's other son, created healing temples where music and other arts were used to treat all manner of illness.

More stories involving music come from the Bible. It is there that angels and harps became linked. God often instructed, either directly or through His emissaries, that His people should use music to achieve their ends and offer Him praise. The last Psalm advises to "Praise God… with the sound of the trumpet, praise

21

Him with the harp and lyre..." The future was even foretold by music, as the ancient Hebrew prophets related their predictions by chanting.

Music is mentioned many times in Revelations. Angels signal with trumpets the devastations that will occur, and the elders sing during the revelation of what is to happen to mankind. A dire warning comes when Babylon's destruction is depicted: "... the great city of Babylon will be thrown down, never to be found again. The music of harpists and musicians, flute players and trumpeters, will never be heard in you again."

An ancient Chinese emperor, Shun, would have agreed that it would have been a terrible curse to have no music. In the second month of every year, he set out on a journey to check on his kingdom. He had to make sure that all was right in the land. But Emperor Shun measured the state of his union not by census figures or taxes collected, or even the standard of living of his subjects.

The Emperor traveled to each region of his land, measuring its condition by testing the exact pitches of its musical notes. He made certain that the five musical notes in the ancient Chinese scale were at the exact same pitch in all of the regions. If the regions differed in their tunings, he felt that they would become separated. If the music was not unified, then the land was not unified.

As for the music itself, its content was just as important. The emperor listened carefully to the kinds of songs being sung. He knew that if the songs were vulgar or profane, the decline of his kingdom's morality was not far behind. Shun would not have been at all surprised to learn of the havoc created by certain music in Greece nearly twenty-five hundred years ago.

About the time of Pericles, when Greek art and civilization were at their peak, a new music emerged. Deviating wildly from its pure, classical form, the music became inharmonic, overmodulated, and rebellious. Over a period of only about twenty years—despite warnings by traditional musicians, scholars, and others—the new music took hold.

It rocked the very foundations of the society, culminating in a political revolution. After the revolution of 404 BC, the musical rebels became even more blatant and crude, writing lyrics that seem eerily similar to some of today's modern songs:

> "I do not sing the old things
> Because the new are the winners.
> Zeus the young is king today;
> Once it was Cronos ruling.
> Go to hell, old dame Music."

by Timotheus of Miletus

It wasn't long until Greece faded as a world power; its position usurped by the Romans. It will be interesting to see if current trends in music have any less devastating an efffect on modern society.

---

*"Words are wonderful enough;*
*but music is even more powerful.*
*It speaks not to our thoughts as words do;*
*it speaks straight to our hearts and spirits;*
*to the very core and root of our souls."*

*Charles Kingsley*

---

We think that the most profound thing that sets us apart from animals is the fact that we can speak. But words and language were not automatically ours. Language developed slowly in humankind. Our human ears have thousands of tiny hairs in the inner ear, called cilia. Researchers have found that about two thirds of the cilia respond and resonate only to *musical* frequencies. That probably means that early man evolved in a state where communication was done primarily through the use of song and music.

Some researchers believe that at one time there was a universal alphabet. It consisted of only two or three tones plus rhythmic patterns that everyone in the world could understand. Think of how you call a pet or child: BOB-by, SU-sie, FLUF-fy. The lilting, sing-song way of using the language is as much a part of the meaning as the words themselves.

Another interesting fact is that almost everyone in the world recognizes a three note sequence like that which starts *"Ring Around the Rosie"* or *"Twinkle, Twinkle Little Star."* Do you remember the series of notes that those who encountered the aliens hummed in the movie *"Close Encounters of the Third Kind?"* The scientists who later tried to communicate with the aliens used those notes, and got a reply. It seems to us that if there is such a thing as a universal language, it would be musical notes.

Even after spoken language became relatively sophisticated, there seemed to be a need for further communication. Words were just not enough for humans to adequately give expression to their deepest, most heartfelt thoughts and emotions. Think of how many times a song has been used to express something that couldn't be said in words.

Minstrels who traveled throughout ancient lands spread the news with their songs. In times when most people could not read or write, these entertainers were the only source of information about the outside world, and people remembered what was said, because it was in song. With a little musical and poetic embellishment, history was recorded for generations to come.

And so it was that music gave an added dimension to communication, the rites of passage, and the ceremonies that ancient man developed to make his society civilized. Music, chanting, dancing, and ritual were all very important for the natives of this and many other lands.

From birth to death, for pauper or prince, music accompanied life.

## A Musical Connection to God

*"Music comes from heaven,*
*rites are shaped by earthly designs"*

*the ancient texts of the Li chi*

While music was definitely an asset for ritual enhancement and communication, it's power to connect humans directly with God was even more important to ancient man. In the pyramids of Egypt there are carvings of musicians playing harps and flutes. Dancers are depicted as well, usually in relation to some kind of ceremony or ritual. Ancient petroglyphs on the walls of caves throughout the world depict flutes and drums being played during ceremonies. Besides the shamans or priests, spirit entities were often pictured in this ancient art.

Given the proliferation of this ritualized art, it seems likely that these civilizations considered music essential to connecting with the spirit world. And, since nothing was more important in

25

many cultures than the connection to Spirit, it would follow that music played an essential role in their lives.

This musical connection to God or the Creator was evident in civilizations around the world. Chanting, one of the most enduring forms of musical expression, is steeped in the sacred. Whether it was a Tibetan monk singing two, or three pitches at once, a yogi intoning "OM," or a Native American singing a three note tune under the stars, chant provided a direct link to the source of All That Is.

---

*"Hear, O my son, the words of the Lord, and incline thy heart's ear."*

*opening words,*
*The Rule of Saint Benedict*

---

Even today, the chants of the Benedictine and Tibetan monks are very popular. No matter what our background—Christian, Buddhist, Native American—we have all heard chant. It inspires a feeling of reverence. We believe that this reverence arises from the profound sense chant gives us, of being connected to something which is greater than ourselves.

We all need to feel that there's something more. We need to know that there is something beyond that which we see and feel every day. We need to feel a connection to the All That Is, for that connection is what nurtures our sense of purpose and self.

But music was not solely for the praise of God or to foster a connection to Him. Countless wars have been fought in the name of God, and much stirring music has been written to spur soldiers on into battle, in His name.

For the knights in the crusades, it was music glorifying God and the Holy Catholic Church that fortified their spirits. When primitive warriors prepared for battle, dancing, drumming, and singing to the Great Spirit was just as important to insure victory as preparing weapons and battle plans.

Even relatively modern songs such as *"Onward Christian Soldiers"* or *"The Battle Hymn of the Republic"* depict the struggle to save souls as a war fought in the name of God.

From the chants of ancient Hebrews enslaved in Egypt, to the Spirituals intoned by Africans brought to America to work the cotton fields, music has been a call to God for deliverance. While music may not have made their plight any better, it did give the downtrodden a connection to their God, and a way to pray continuously for aid. It was a way to vent their fear, isolation, and sorrow.

Have you ever been to a service in a southern Baptist church? If so, you will never forget the energy coming through the powerful music that is such an integral part of the service. Ecstasy, praise, and the love of God permeates every cell in your body during such a service. In that experience, you can have no doubt that music is a direct line to the Creator.

## Music Today and Tomorrow

Unfortunately, the powerful musical connection to each other and the cosmos was mostly lost in modern Western society. With the advent of medical institutions, pharmaceutical companies, and psychotherapy, music was relegated to the history books—a quaint therapy practiced by witch doctors and voodoo chiefs. Its status, and that of the people who made music, fell from exalted to tolerated. With few exceptions, music was demoted, in a way, to nothing more than entertainment. While its power was largely ignored by the medical and psychological establishments of modern times, music did not stop influencing people or reflecting their emotions and lives.

Think of the songs of the 1960s—flower power and peace and love. Songs such as *"Blowin' in the Wind"*[1] and *"What the World Needs Now, is Love, Sweet Love"*[2] clashed with the Bay of Pigs and the Vietnam War. The mantra of the times was "peace," expressed through music, but the country was at war. The confusion of the music mirrored the confusion of the times. War, peace, love, fear. Everything was thrown at this generation, and it was reflected in the music.

Look at music today. How much more could it possibly typify the society in which we live? Gangster Rap blares from a car stereo right next to an SUV playing the Doors. Christian Rock has gained popularity alongside New Age music. Our music is as diverse as our society.

And so, while government doesn't formally acknowledge music as a force in society, and is cutting music out of that most important of society's realms—the public schools—music does indeed shape our lives. If we are to be physically and spiritually healthy, we must carefully consider exactly what kind of music we are allowing into our lives.

Later we'll be talking more about how negative music affects us, but the important thing to remember is that we can control what we hear. We can encourage our medical establishments, the education system, and even corporate America to program positive music into our living and working space.

---

[1] Blowin' in the Wind, Bob Dylan, 1962, ©Warner Bros., Inc
[2] What the World Needs Now, is Love, Sweet Love, David and Bacharach, 1965, © Casa David and New Hidden Valley Music

Music was used for centuries to keep cultures whole, intact, and powerful. The health of a society was monitored and kept intact by the power of music. It can be used that way again, leading to healthy individuals and a modern culture that is at peace.

---

*"… the first duty of music is to complement and enhance life."*

Carlos Santana

---

♫ *Music
creates order
out of chaos.*

*Yehudi Menuhin* ♪

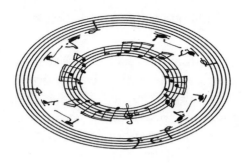

# TWO

# Music — The Art of Vibration

*"No musical vibrations are ever lost...*
*they will go on vibrating through the cosmos*
*for eternity."*

*Joscelyn Godwin 1991*

Every material thing—every person, animal, rock, and tree on the earth, even Mother Earth herself—has its own natural resonating frequency. The Earth's electromagnetic field, deep space, and people in a meditative state, are all resonating at a frequency of approximately 7.8 hertz. It is called the Schumann Resonating Frequency.

Every cell in every person, rock, and tree also has its own natural resonating frequency which is ideally in harmony with the unit as a whole. Every sound, from the delicacy of a pure musical note to the harsh retort of a gun, sends out a wave of energy. This wave is vibrating at its own frequency, which then affects everything in its path.

In human beings, the balanced interaction of all the frequencies resonating in and through our bodies is what makes us work. When our frequencies resonate in sync, we are healthy. We feel good, and we feel connected with our own selves and those around us. We are "in tune."

For whales and dolphins, resonating in perfect harmony is essential. If these creatures are not in tune with each other, they cannot communicate. Reproduction and survival depend completely upon this ability to recognize and reply to each other's "song."

For humans, the issue is not quite so critical, but when we are out of tune, many problems can develop. Just as all the musicians in a symphony orchestra must be tuned to each other for the music to sound good, so, too, must all of our cells be in tune with each other for us to feel good. And just as any number of things can make a musical instrument go out of tune—like changes in temperature, humidity or a sudden bump—any number of things can jostle the cells in our body out of tune.

A good example of the physical effect of vibrating energy is the scraping of fingernails against a chalkboard. This grating noise produces physical changes in anyone who hears it. Our teeth tingle and the hair on the back of our neck stands up. The tone itself is creating a frequency that is adversely affecting the rate of vibration in the cells of the body experiencing it.

Have you ever used an ultrasonic machine to repel rodents or insects? These devices work on pure sound. Their frequencies produce sound that only the pests can hear, but it is absolutely repelling to them. It creates a very definite physical reaction and they scurry away.

Isn't that how you feel when you hear unpleasant sounds? You try to get away. If you can't get away, your body reacts negatively to those sounds. We notice the most obvious things at once—we cover our ears, tense up, or start to get nervous. But the effects go far beyond the obvious.

Scientific tests have shown that bombardment of the body by unpleasant sounds actually increases blood pressure, pulse, and respiratory rates. The blood's magnesium level falls and extra fats are released into the bloodstream.

Music is a way to experience vibrations in a pure form. Music is the art of vibrations. Whether it has a positive or negative physical effect depends on how it is arranged and presented. The source of the sound, the volume, even the purity of the tone, has everything to do with the physical effect it has on our human bodies and other living things.

## Good Vibrations for Plants

Everyone has heard the stories of miraculous recoveries of houseplants which have had music played near them. You may even have tried playing Mozart for your own philodendron. It makes a lot of sense, if you understand that everything has its own natural resonating frequency, and that different musical frequencies have varying effects on all things. Scientific research has confirmed this fact, especially for plants.

A researcher in Minnesota found that agricultural plants, including corn, responded and grew at an amazing rate when they were exposed to the sounds of the sitar (a traditional stringed instrument from India).

Another researcher, in Denver, Colorado, compared the effects that different kinds of music had on plants. We found this research very interesting.

Plants were placed in five identical greenhouses. Soil, light, and water conditions were all identical, and the types of plants were the same in all of the greenhouses. For several months, the researcher pumped different kinds of music into each of the greenhouses: in the first, Bach was played; in the second, Indian music; the third, loud rock; and the fourth, country and western music. In the fifth greenhouse, no music was played at all.

The plants in the greenhouse where only loud rock was played did not do well at all. Their growth was stunted and they would not flower. In the greenhouses with Bach and Indian music, the plants were green and healthy, with many flowers. The plants who heard country and western music grew the same as those with no music, at a moderate rate with a normal amount of flowers.

It doesn't seem likely that the plants had an emotional response to the music; it must have been something in the actual rate of vibration, the frequency of the soundwaves that affected their growth. If music has such a profound effect on relatively simple organisms, what must it do to more complex systems?

*"By means of sound it is possible to cause geometric figures to form on sand, and also to cause objects to be shattered. How much more powerful, then, must be the impact of this force on the vibrating, living substance of our sensitive bodies."*

*Roberto Assagioli, M.D.*

## Order and Disorder

You can actually see the effects that various sounds have on other substances. Set a large glass of water near a stereo speaker. Turn the music on and see how it moves the water. If you have a chance, visit a discovery-type museum. There are usually displays which allow you to experiment with sound, and you can see its effect on substances such as sand sprinkled on a drum head, or sawdust or shavings on a saw or piece of metal. As the materials are exposed to different kinds of sounds—music, sawing, etc.—they take on different patterns, because the different frequencies, or lengths of the sound waves, are affecting these substances in their own way.

A famous researcher, Hans Jenny, studied these formations carefully. He took many photographs of beautiful, symmetrical shapes which were formed by powders vibrating on a surface that was vibrating with sound, especially music. He demonstrated and recorded visually the fact that sound produces order out of randomness. But what if sound produces disorder?

We've all heard of people being able to sing a note which breaks glass. When a jet bursts through the sound barrier, it causes a sonic boom that breaks windows for miles around. That is what happens when sounds create disorder on a visible scale. Now think about the disorder all those vibrations are creating inside our bodies, where we cannot see their effects.

## Sound and the Human Body

Consider all of the sounds that you hear every day. The jangling of an alarm clock, airplanes flying overhead, trucks and buses rumbling by, the loud music coming from megabass speakers in the car next to you at the stoplight. Televisions, telephones, dogs barking, children playing, sirens, machinery at work. Just imagine all the different frequencies that those sounds are emitting.

Now think of all the frequencies you cannot hear. The human ear has a very limited range of hearing. Sound waves above and below that range are not physically heard, but they still affect the rate of resonance in our bodies. One example of inaudible sound is the radio wave. These tones are audible only when you have a receiver with which to pick them up, but they are always there. Hundreds of thousands of them are entering and bombarding our bodies and individual cells every second, every minute, every day for our entire lives. The trouble is, many of these frequencies are damaging to the human body. They are literally altering the natural resonance of our DNA and changing our cellular structures.

If you have ten tuning forks all tuned to the same frequency, and you strike one, they will all begin to resonate together. However, if you strike a tuning fork tuned differently, and place it near the others, they will all stop. Now, if these dissonant frequencies can stop the vibration of a simple tuning fork, what must they do to the delicate balance in our human bodies?

To begin with, they can physically damage our ears. People in modern society have a great degree of hearing loss. Whether frequencies originate from random noise like jet engines or rock music emanating from stacks of amplifiers, the vibrations actually damage the delicate tissues which allow us to hear.

The physical damage, however, is dwarfed by the social consequences of hearing loss. Conversations become difficult, movies are not nearly so enjoyable, even driving takes on an added dimension of danger. Many people who suffer from hearing loss become despondent and withdrawn, just because it's too hard to communicate.

The ears are not the only part of the body which suffer from jarring, loud, or discordant sounds, including certain kinds of music. When exposed to a multitude of instruments and voices, an erratic beat, and electronic distortion of the notes themselves, the resonating frequency of the human body is thrown into chaos. The organs begin to vibrate out of sync with the nervous system, which can't keep up with the rate of breathing, which in turn effects the entire organism.

Is it any wonder that so many of us feel stressed, tired, and irritable? Our cells are vibrating at erratic levels, out of sync with each other. In advanced cases, this bombardment of frequencies can cause many physical changes and lead to disease in the body. How do you counteract this insidious invasion by sound?

You do this by being conscious of frequencies that disrupt your body's own rate of resonance, eliminating them, and ultimately replacing them with frequencies that have a positive impact on the body.

*"For there is music wherever there is
harmony, order or proportion.
And thus far we may maintain
the music of the sphere."*

Sir Thomas Browne

## Balancing Your Body's Frequencies

There are many therapists who use tone generators and sound wave machines to help people get their bodies vibrating at their optimum rates. You could try that approach, but it may be very expensive and not readily available where you live. What other options do you have?

The easiest and most enjoyable thing is MUSIC. Technically, music is no more than a series of notes or tones arranged in a mathematically precise and aesthetically pleasing pattern. Tones are just some of the dozens of sounds traveling through the air, water, or solid objects at any given time. Whether we hear them or not, these tones resonate through us constantly.

If you want to change the resonating frequency of your body, listening to or making music is very powerful. Listening to the soothing tones of chant, Native American flute, harp, or synthesized strings is a great way to get the body resonating back to its proper, natural state.

Sit quietly in a comfortable chair, and really listen to *"Millennium,"* the CD that's included with this book. We've included this music because it is pure. The melodies are simple, the arrangements uncomplicated. You can listen to each instrument and feel its impact on your physical body.

This experience is enhanced if you wear padded headphones that cover the whole ear, because then you get the full effect of all of the frequencies in the music. Also, it blocks out other audible sounds that could be creating discordance. Close your eyes. Keep out all sensory input but for this music.

Each tune has a different range of frequencies, different melodies, and they will give you different physical responses. Allow your body to respond to the frequencies. Close your eyes and breathe deeply. Pay attention to how your physical body changes. Immediately it will be more relaxed. There will be a difference in your blood pressure, your heartrate, your breathing.

Once your body is calm—resonating at a more balanced frequency—you will be amazed at how different things look. Situations that might have bothered you, people who may have annoyed you, just won't matter as much. You'll have so much more freedom to think your own thoughts and feel your true feelings because they won't be governed by energies over which you have no control.

Another excellent way to calm down the physical body is to listen to a pure beat. Any repetitive sound, such as a metronome, a heartbeat, or constant, even drumming, has a regulating effect on the biological functioning of the human body. Go to a music store and get an old-fashioned wooden metronome. Set it on "largo," about 40 beats per minute. This slow, soothing rhythm has an hypnotic effect. After ten minutes or so, you will find yourself in a very relaxed state. Even the ticking of an old-fashioned grandfather clock can have the effect of regulating your body.

Whenever you're feeling over-stimulated or irritated, stop. Analyze what's bothering you. You'll be amazed at how often it is a sound—music, machinery, perhaps voices. If you can't eliminate the noise or get away from it, at least you will recognize that it is noise that's making you feel stressed or upset, and not some unknown element.

You can counteract noise overload by humming. If you have to travel on a subway or bus, or even in your car, or if you work in a factory with loud machinery, you can help your body resonate at its optimum rate by humming. You don't have to hum loud enough for anyone else to hear, just loud enough to feel it in your own body. As you hum, you will find yourself making tones that make your body feel more comfortable, and the noise from which you cannot escape will not bother you as much. Give it a try.

*"No one may enter*
*who does not know earth's rhythm"*

*inscription over the entrance to*
*Plato's academy in Athens*

We know that every individual body and every thing is being bombarded by sound and noise. Consider the dissonance created by the overwhelming number of frequencies penetrating everyone on Earth. Nothing is in tune with anything else.

Is it any wonder that there is so much anger, mistrust, and fear? How are you supposed to relate to and communicate with each other under these sound stresses? What if we could somehow balance and synchronize ourselves with each other and the planet? It makes perfect sense that communication would be much easier and we would all feel much healthier and more peaceful.

Barbara Marx Hubbard is a futurist who believes that we could all benefit by humming a certain note. She believes that D flat is the note that most closely matches the resonating frequency of the earth. She feels that, if enough people were to hum or otherwise create this tone together, it would counteract the discordant frequencies racing around the planet, and raise the consciousness of Mother Earth and the people inhabiting her.

It makes sense to us, and we would dearly love to see what would happen if several million people hummed that tone at the same time. Would it be like the walls of Jericho tumbling down? Would the walls of fear and mistrust crumble, allowing all of us to love and understand each other?

There are recordings which have the resonating frequency of the earth encoded in them. A wonderful example is Dean Evenson's *"Ocean Dreams."* Combined with pure music and natural effects—such as ocean waves and dolphin and whale song—these frequencies have an incredible impact on our bodies. They put us back into tune with the earth herself.

If we could all balance our frequencies with each other, the earth, and the universe, we would have an actual physical connection via sound. Just imagine what it would be like here on this beautiful Earth without conflicting sound energy. Wouldn't it be wonderful if the whole planet was in tune?

*In every note there is hope.*
*In every musical phrase,*
*there is healing,*
*and in every song,*
*joy.*
*Music offers a solution*
*for every person;*
*perhaps for every illness, too.*

*Cathy Kunkel*

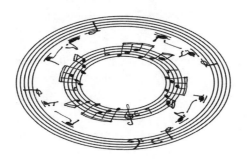

# THREE

# Music as Medicine

*"… seek out a man who is skillful in playing
the harp;
and when the evil spirit is upon you,
he will play it and you will be well."*

*Samuel 16:14–16*

There is evidence that musical healing began over thirty thousand years ago. Even though sickness was a mystery to the ancient peoples, they knew intuitively that sound was essential to recovery. In those earliest days, simple tones and mono-syllabic chants were the sounds used to cure all manner of illnesses.

As their communities became more organized, the health of each member became increasingly important. The community's existence was dependent on hunting and gathering, and each individual had a specific task that had to be done daily. A sick tribesman was a threat to the survival of the group. He had to be made well as quickly as possible. And just as the health of the community depended on its individual members, each of the members depended upon the community for their personal health.

The whole community helped in the healing process. Someone would gather herbs and make elixirs and potions, while others would start fires over which the medicines would be infused. Special healing huts or areas would be prepared, and the sick person would be brought there and tended by family. Then the shaman would come in and the healing would begin. The spiritual forces were invoked to make this person well; called upon mostly by the chanting and drumming that was their sacred music.

As we proceed in time, the details of how music was used to cure illness become much clearer. Ten thousand years ago, the ancient Egyptians and Sumerians successfully treated cancers with specific tones. In the Talmud, a specific song was recommended to protect oneself from epidemics, and the early Christians sang psalms for healing.

It was generally believed that evil spirits were the cause of most physical ailments. Medicine men (and women) and shamans in all indigenous cultures used music to coax evil spirits out of the afflicted. Perhaps the most famous incident of this kind is the

Biblical story of David playing his harp to relieve King Saul of his evil spirit.

The ancient Chinese felt that a single note could create good or evil in individuals or in the universe, depending upon the will of the musician. It was therefore imperative that anyone using music in healing practices be sincere and honest.

Today we can see living examples of the work of shamans in indigenous tribes around the world. Sometimes called witch-doctors, these healers use drumming, chanting, dancing, and singing to chase out evil spirits, reestablish the good spirits, and heal their tribesmen and women. These time-tested techniques have worked for people for thousands of years, but many Westerners scoff at them.

## Modern Medicine

Today, the health of one individual rarely has any affect on the community as a whole. Unless the sick person is a head of state, his or her health is of no concern to us. And even if the president of the country is sick, it has no lasting effect on us. A whole city won't collapse and die of hunger because there is one less CEO. There is no longer a connection between the survival of a community and the health of specific individuals within it.

In our highly compartmentalized society, only rigorously tested techniques and drugs administered by a few highly-trained individuals, are used on the sick. They are governed by insurance companies and the threat of malpractice suits. Very little of the patient's emotional and spiritual life is even considered in the modern hospital. Family members are allowed to visit only under strict guidelines and are not allowed to actively participate in the treatment process.

White walls and sheets. Monitors and sterilized instruments. Antibiotics and urine samples. Aspirins that cost twenty dollars each. Five minute, three hundred dollar visits with a specialist who would never recognize you on the street. Hospital food! These are the images of a modern medical facility. It is understandable that people are terrified of the medical system. It's no wonder they want to get out of hospitals as quickly as possible and often heal much faster when they do.

What's missing? What's been lost in this quest for scientific treatment of all illness? Spirituality. Intuition. Family. Music. These powerful healers have been tossed to the wayside by modern medicine. There is no proof, scientists say, that anything but surgery, certain approved therapies, and drugs can cure illness.

While they're in the hospital, patients are trying to recover from major trauma and illness. But what is bombarding their senses while they're there? The beeping of monitors, crackling of loudspeakers, and calls of "Code Blue." How are you supposed to get better with all that going on? It truly is a wonder anyone can recuperate in such an environment.

So much of that which is essential to the human condition is neglected by the billion dollar, profit-driven industry with which we entrust our lives. We recently approached a hospital in Las Vegas about playing for patients in a cancer ward. The hospital would not even entertain the notion of us entering the ward because of its concern for patient confidentiality. How sad that a truly beneficial, healing therapy was denied because of their lawyer's opinion. Instead of healing harp music, chemotherapy patients were being subjected to the dramas of a television soap opera.

## Healing the Whole Person

Healing is about so much more than medicine and surgery. What about the Chinese and Native American herbal medicines? What about diet, music and tone therapy, and meditation? What about the love of family, the support of friends? What about laughter? What about prayer?

Your physical health is intertwined with your emotional and spiritual well-being. Do not entrust it blindly to drugs and surgeries. Of course, we would never suggest that you not go to a doctor or submit to surgery to remove a cancerous tumor. However, know this: *everything that modern medicine offers you is not everything there is.*

In addition to the various holistic practices scattered throughout the country, in some hospitals where brave and far-thinking administrators have seen the benefits of music in action, change is on the horizon.

In an effort to minimize the negative impact of hospital sounds, comforting, instrumental music is being played in some cancer wards, intensive care units, and therapy centers. The effect is to make patients more comfortable, less stressed, and happier. It also makes their bodies resonate at a healthier rate.

Thanks to the work of modern music therapists, healing musicians, and anthropologists who bring back to us the healing techniques of other cultures (and our own history), music is beginning once again to be recognized as having a value above and beyond entertainment. The imaginative, intuitive practices of shamans are being examined, and music therapists are beginning to incorporate more of them into their own therapies. The value of spiritual connectedness and intuitive feeling is slowly being accepted by some scientifically trained western healers.

Just as alternative therapies such as acupuncture and chiropractic are being covered by medical insurance and prescribed by western doctors, with enough pressure and proof, music could also become an accepted part of treatment for any number of diseases.

We've only just begun to rediscover how powerful music is in the treatment of almost every illness known to man. What we're offering you here is a mere sampling of the wonderful ways that music is helping cure or alleviate some of our most common maladies.

> "Each illness has a musical solution.
> The shorter and more complete the solution—
> the greater the musical talent of the physician.
> Sickness demands manifold solutions.
> The selection of the most appropriate solution
> determines the talent of the physician."
>
> Novalis

When we speak here of physically healing music, we would like to stress that the range and frequencies of the music being used is very important. While some classical and even pop music is valuable, the true healing of the human body comes not from complicated melodies, harmonic interludes, or lush arrangements. Our bodies have a rhythm like the earth herself, and if we tap into those rhythms and sounds, music healing is much more effective.

Imagine the roar of the ocean, the rustling of the wind, the drone of insects. All of these are naturally occurring frequencies that our bodies already know how to use to regain balance. When music is added for healing, it must be steady, uncomplicated, and pure. To fully utilize the innate healing abilities of the body, we have to let it recognize and assimilate the different natural tones that are being given to it. Music with a constant, steady rhythm, and a kind of drone, is especially valuable. We'll give examples at the end of the chapter, but it is most important to remember this: constant tempos, simple melodies that repeat with regularity, and lots of space for the natural frequencies to get through are very important.

Additionally, the music itself must be something you enjoy. It must be pleasing to you; otherwise, it will either have no beneficial effect, or it could actually aggravate your condition. Take time to listen to various recordings when you go to a music store. Listen carefully, allowing yourself time to really feel the music. Your body will tell you what is best for it. We've included listening techniques in Chapter Ten. Use them when you're choosing music, because they will help you recognize what effect particular music has on you. You can then analyze what is best for your particular situation.

Our final goal in this book is to help you achieve physical, spiritual, and emotional health. While modern medicine is valuable, indeed, don't forget that your true, whole, and healthy self depends on balance and inner peace. Music is one of the most powerful tools you can use to achieve this ideal.

## Music and the Immune System

From AIDS to Chronic Fatigue Syndrome to cancer, it is the inability of our immune system to fight off attacks which allows disease to take hold in our bodies. To be healthy, we must strengthen our immune system, and music is an excellent way to do that.

There is no question that there is a connection between what we ingest, what we hear, what we feel, and the way our immune system operates. There are many stresses put upon us by our environment: new strains of bacteria; food additives and hormones; air, water, and noise pollution; and frequency pollution. All of these things tax our immune systems to a dangerous degree.

Damaging frequencies enter our bodies on a daily basis. Many frequencies we can hear, but the most damaging may, in fact, be those that we cannot hear. It's more than just power lines emitting electromagnetic radiation. Television, radio, and military communications, even air traffic control signals are slicing the very air we breathe, altering and re-programming the cells in our bodies. Recently, there have been reports about how microwave radiation produced by cellular telephones may be instrumental in the development of brain tumors. In the workplace, people who sit in front of computer monitors all day face increased threats of cancer. We don't even know if it's safe to stand near your microwave oven.

The fact is, we just don't know enough about any of these new kinds of potentially lethal frequencies. They've only been around for the last seventy-five years. What we do know, is that people are dying from cancer, AIDS, neuromuscular diseases, even bacterial infections, at alarming rates. This is despite the fact that hundreds of millions of dollars are spent every year finding cures for these diseases. Are our immune systems being stressed too much? Can music help?

Clinical researcher, Dr. Theodore A Baroody, Jr, author of *"Alkalize or Die,"* has found that discordant (acidic) sound actually disrupts our basic organ function and causes eruptions of enzymes and hormones. This leads to the actual destruction of cells, which weakens our immune system, leaving the door open to disease.

While music itself does not produce damaging electromagnetic waves, certain kinds of music and other discordant sounds certainly can emit frequencies which produce "acid" in our systems. Therefore, we have to choose music which will counteract both the heard and unheard sounds that wreak havoc on our immune systems.

Dr. Baroody claims that there is "acid" and "alkaline" music. Acid-producing music is that such as hard rock and rap— anything that makes you feel angry, confused, jumpy, or scattered. Alkaline producing music is soft classical, ambient instrumental, meditative—anything that makes you feel relaxed, content, happy.

Harmonious sound, including alkaline music, relaxes and synchronizes our nerves, organs and the glandular system. This purely physical effect is only part of the way the right kind of music strengthens our immune system. Preliminary studies show that music stimulates the immune system by capturing the ebb and flow of emotional tides in the body. While one piece of music can bring about a sudden burst of tears... another can trigger laughter and happiness. Music strengthens us physically and emotionally. It gives us peace and hope and love, and more than anything, we need those very human qualities to keep our immune systems healthy.

## Heart Disease

How many people do you know who have suffered a heart attack? How many have survived one only to have another heart attack later that kills them? They may have been taking medication, following diet and exercise programs, and still their hearts gave out.

It is an absolute fact that the right kind of music—like harp music—decreases stress. Stress is a major factor in heart disease. Music, then, should be a natural addition to any course of treatment for heart attack victims. Unfortunately, that is not generally the case. Have you ever heard a doctor prescribe moderate exercise, a healthy diet, and regular exposure to soothing music?

Well, we're prescribing it here. In Chapter Five, we've set out a whole series of relaxation techniques, meditations, and suggested music selections which reduce stress. They should be used daily, just as the pills and other treatments a doctor would recommend. The evidence of the power of music to aid recovery from heart attacks is not just anecdotal. There are scientific studies which prove it. When Saint Joseph Hospital in New York City installed a music listening system in its intensive care unit, the death rate for heart attack patients in their ward dropped dramatically. Eight to twelve percent fewer patients died in this unit as compared to the national average.

Imagine the feeling. You're in pain, you're frightened, possibly dying. You're rushed into an emergency room. There are monitors beeping and pulsing, crash carts are being wheeled from room to room, doctors and nurses are running through the halls, the public address system is calling doctors' names every few seconds. How are you ever to feel better with all this commotion going on around you?

A critical care nurse from Dallas, Texas, Cathie Guzzetta, watched helplessly for years as frightened patients passed through her ward. She decided to try music and relaxation techniques on them, with great success. Later, in a formal study in Washington, D.C., she found that using music therapy and teaching patients relaxation techniques lowered heart rates and reduced blood pressure. People who had never relaxed before learned to use music, muscle relaxation, and meditation to feel better and reduce their chances of having another attack. Once these individuals learned how to listen to and let music help them settle down, they experienced great comfort in their newfound abilities to relax.

Of course, whenever you have heart problems, you should consult a physician. But you have to realize that a doctor does not have music in the accepted list of treatments for angina or mitral valve prolapse. Medical schools just don't teach prospective doctors about the amazing power of music to heal. Don't discount its power to heal an ailing heart just because music is not in the medical books.

## High Blood Pressure

Despite all manner of drugs, health clubs, and cholesterol- and fat-free foods, nearly forty million Americans suffer from high blood pressure. How can that be?

It's because we are a nation of over-achievers, bent on conquering each other and the world. That mindset can lead to only one thing—stress. And from stress flows high blood pressure and its related problems including strokes and heart attacks.

The right kind of music is a powerful antidote to the stresses that raise our blood pressure. By incorporating relaxation techniques and meditation with the music listening experience, you can see a dramatic decrease in blood pressure.

However, the music must be devoid of anything that creates fear or recalls painful memories. It's also important that the music be simple, calming, and have a consistent tempo. Complicated jazz, heavy rock, and passionate classical pieces are definitely not appropriate. Instrumental, ambient, or meditative music is best.

Music is also a wonderful reinforcement for the lifestyle changes that are so important in controlling blood pressure. Exercise is much more enjoyable and easier to manage if it is synchronized to music. Another powerful lifestyle change is to learn to play an instrument or to sing. The energy created by making music is a powerful blood pressure regulator.

## Stroke

One of the most common results of high blood pressure is a stroke. Ideally, music therapy should be started well in advance of a stroke occurring, but if one does strike, music is of immense help in rehabilitation.

Depression is a common hurdle over which many stroke patients must leap. It's very easy to feel sorry for yourself when talking, walking, perhaps even eating, has become difficult or impossible. In a study in Scotland, researchers found that hospitalized patients who received music therapy in conjunction with their other treatments were far less likely to suffer depression. They were much more positive in their outlook and had fewer episodes of anxiety.

There is much more help that music can give to the stroke patient. Imagine yourself trying to learn to walk again after a severe stroke. How difficult it is to send the messages from your brain to your leg and have it do what you're asking. What if your brain had a little help? What if music was introduced which helped your body remember the movements? What about some music that you used to dance to? Maybe a good old-fashioned Strauss waltz, or how about some disco beat? Anything that makes you remember dancing is perfect. It should be happy and should encourage positive memories. But more importantly, it will stimulate the automatic response to move the feet and legs.

Another interesting use of beat and music was used by researchers in Colorado. They imbedded rhythms provided by metronome pulses into music that patients enjoyed. This rhythmic stimulation actually helped the patients improve their foot placement, helped them stride more evenly, and increased their ability to continue walking over periods of time. Best of all, even when the patients no longer had this stimulation, the walking patterns learned with the aid of this rhythmic device continued. In other words, they did not relapse or develop ungainly patterns of walking.

Many stroke patients lose the use of an arm. Imagine the benefits of playing a piano or beating on a drum. Beating a drum along with a therapist or a piece of recorded music helps establish a pattern in the mind and in the body. In addition to strengthening the limb, it makes more sense than just opening and closing a hand or moving an arm up and down. The rhythmic motion helps the limb remember the correct way to move long after the drumming is discontinued.

And what about talking? For many stroke patients, it is very difficult to form words and sentences. Many even lose their voices completely, for a time. Humming and toning are marvelous tools to exercise the vocal chords and to send vibrations throughout the body. These vibrations stimulate the body's own healing mechanism. Soon it becomes easier to develop words and sentences and to establish a cadence that makes it easier to communicate.

Therapists are only beginning to experiment with sound and music for stroke patients. Even if the therapies being offered to you or a loved one do not include music, experiment yourself. Play music during the walking exercises. Sing, hum, bang on a drum. It can't hurt, and you may just find a miracle in the making.

## Cancer

A German study by Dr. Ralph Spintge indicates that musicians have a significantly lower rate of cancer than the general population. As musicians, we're delighted to know that. The question is, why musicians? Is it purely cellular? Is it emotional?

We have cancer cells in our bodies all of the time. The trick is to make sure they don't grow into something that will kill us. Since music stimulates the immune system, it may prevent the cancer cells from grabbing hold, mutating, and invading the body.

But the power of music is more than just stimulating the immune system. Research has shown that certain musical tones can actually reduce the size of existing tumors and make cancer cells disappear.

A French musician, Fabien Maman, has been working with Helene Grimal, a researcher in Paris. Together they exposed cancer cells to various tones at various intervals. They found that cancer cells in test tubes would actually begin to disintegrate when exposed to a specific tone for twenty-one minutes.

They were able to test these findings with female patients who had breast tumors. When the afflicted women toned specific notes for periods of twenty-one minutes at a time, for a total of three and a half hours a day, their tumors actually diminished. One of the women had surgery even after tests showed the tumor was shrinking. Amazingly, the tumor itself had reduced in size, had not metastasized, and was easily removed. No cancer returned. The other patients had no surgeries, and demonstrated no further symptoms when the experiment was over.

With a disease like cancer, it seems that the actual vibration, the physical production of a particular frequency or range of frequencies in the body, has an enormous effect on the diseased cells. While listening to music is definitely a positive thing, it may be even more important for cancer patients to actually make music.

In addition to eating whole foods, taking recommended therapies, and exercising, picking up and playing a guitar, an autoharp, an Irish bodhran, or portable keyboard can really help. Native American flutes and your own voice are also wonderful instruments for this purpose. Don't concern yourself with playing structured music... just get close to the instrument and make sound. Select the strings setting on your keyboard and hold down a rich, low note (such as D flat) for a few minutes. Blow a long, soothing note on the flute. Hum.

Find a tone that stimulates the afflicted part of your body. Let your body absorb the vibrations as you focus your attention on the sound waves penetrating the part of the body that needs to be healed. Experiment with different notes. You will feel intuitively which ones are helping. Try toning with your voice, or playing on an instrument, those certain notes for twenty-one minute periods.

While we're not suggesting that you bypass any therapies recommended by your doctor, we believe that you can give yourself a much better chance of conquering cancer by supplementing your treatment with the inclusion of music. In addition, it makes you feel involved in your own recovery, and everyone needs to feel that they're ultimately in charge of their own body.

## Headaches

One of the most common of ailments—the headache. What do you do when you get one? Most people reach for over-the-counter or prescription medications.

There is no question that most headaches come on because of stress. The best way to deal with that, of course, is by relaxation. Learning to consciously relax specific muscles, such as those around your eyes, neck, and face is important. Listening to calming, transportive music diverts your mind away from the pain. Instead of chemicals, music is the "drug" which allows you to relax.

Besides the emotional release that music offers, there are other benefits which are purely physical. The frequency—or rate of vibration of the tones themselves—is the source of pain relief. The vibrations produced by toning are especially helpful. Toning is the production of sounds with your own voice. For some kinds of headaches, producing the proper tones can create a vibration which actually counteracts the source of pain. The trick is to tap into the right frequency.

As with nearly everything in music healing, there is no right or wrong. The tone that makes *your* headache go away is not necessarily the same tone that helps someone else. Remember, it all has to do with natural resonating frequency. You just have to find your own frequency and tap into it. Experiment by making various drawn-out sounds like "ahhhh," "ooooh," "hmmmm," or "ommmm." Tone higher or lower, opening and closing your mouth, shaping it in various ways. Eventually you will find a tone which produces a vibration that feels right to you. You will notice a decrease in the level of pain. See what happens when you tone for five minutes.

Of course, the idea is not to get a headache in the first place. You can prevent headaches, even migraines. Use guided imagery, meditation, and other relaxation techniques in conjunction with music on a regular basis, at least twice a week. We offer wonderful exercises in Chapter Five and Chapter Twelve of this book. If you take the time to pamper yourself a bit, you will see an amazing decrease in the frequency of your headaches

# Chronic Pain

So many people suffer from chronic pain. The source may be anything from injuries received in an automobile accident to a degenerative disc disease. Very little can affect one's life so totally as living with chronic pain. Sleep patterns are disrupted, the ability to think rationally and process information is impeded, and social activities are often curtailed, leaving the sufferer feeling isolated and lonely.

Of course, there are many pain medications available; however, their side effects are often as bad as the problem causing the pain in the first place. Therefore, many alternative health professionals are using acupressure, acupuncture, hypnosis, and other therapies, all with some degree of success.

Music is an enormous boost for all of these therapies. Remember, music is—at its very root—sound. The frequencies created by sound (audible or inaudible) have an immense impact on the body's vibratory rate. By using just the right frequency, sound can actually decrease the body's experienced pain. We're sure you've heard of ultrasound. It is in effect, inaudible sound, and is used extensively in physical therapy to help ease pain and actually heal afflicted tissues.

In addition to its physiological benefits as sound, music is also very powerful in helping chronic sufferers deal psychologically with the pain. They learn to use music to lower the stress associated with pain, and to relax muscles which tense up in reaction to pain. For everything from childbirth to burns, music has helped people detach from the pain and learn to cope with it in a much more positive fashion. Music also helps alter the perception of time, which helps decrease the perceived pain.

For psychologically escaping intense pain, new age or classical music is not necessarily the best therapy. Pop music, folk rock, and other upbeat music is really the best. We're talking about music from the Beach Boys to the Eagles to Sheryl Crow. Music therapists who work with teenage burn victims have found that rock music is most effective. The main thing to understand here is that *any* music can have emotionally therapeutic effects against pain. Use whatever works for you, and remember, it's okay to turn up the volume.

## Arthritis

Musicians suffer from arthritis just like tens of thousands of other people. In fact, when they're not playing, many instrumentalists suffer terrible pain in their hands and fingers. But when they play, they forget about the pain. Playing music is like having your own, internal cortisone factory.

Other than the obvious aesthetic joy of creating music, the actual physical act of playing, of moving the fingers, is therapeutic. If you don't move arthritic joints, they become stiff and useless. So our first suggestion if you have arthritis is to *use those joints*. Get a portable piano or keyboard. Play the xylophone. Beat gently on a drum.

You are probably aware that there are various kinds of arthritis. The kind that attacks many people as they get older is rheumatoid arthritis. With this particular disease, guided imagery and music are especially helpful. By imagining themselves moving about freely, without pain, sufferers who listen to music can actually reduce pain and swelling, and move about much more easily. Additionally, they are happier and better able emotionally to deal with pain and the limitations of the disease itself.

The kind of music is important here. Anything with words is not as effective as instrumentals. Classical music seems to stimulate the healing process, as does new age music with the sounds of nature in the background. Instrumental music allows you to imagine freely. The music is a conduit to travel in your mind to a place that is healing. To imagine oneself in beautiful surroundings, healthy and free of pain, is the first step in creating wellness. Magnified many times over by music, this power of the mind *can* and *does* reduce pain, increase the ability to move, and reduce the need for medication.

## Alzheimer's Disease

Alzheimer's Disease is one of the most frightening conditions that the aged face. They are unable to remember people or events, have little or no attention span, and forget how to interact with people. The world becomes mysterious and frightening when there is no past or future. Or perhaps they live only in the past — the present does not exist, and the future cannot be conceived. Some Alzheimer's patients eventually have no way to communicate because there is no frame of reference.

Music therapists and volunteer musicians who work with the aging, confirm that music brings people out of their shells. There are many stories of patients who previously just sat in their wheelchairs, coming to life and clapping and singing along when a favorite tune from their past was played.

Besides offering patients some joy and a chance to sing or dance, music is often a door to communication. Because so often they lapse into what is almost a catatonic state, they don't even speak with people they know. When music that is familiar—music of their youth or a familiar hymn—is played or sung, it's as though a light goes on.

Music is not a magical cure for Alzheimer's. So far, there is no evidence that, once a patient has succumbed to the ravages of the disease, it offers any long-term benefits as far as speech or memory is concerned. However, there is evidence that it may slow the advancement of the worst of the disease by being a memory aid. It can also improve the patient's quality of life, because music can offer a chance for social interaction, communication, and happiness.

Alzheimer's takes an immense toll on anyone who cares for someone with this disease. Whether you are a paid attendant, a spouse, or a child, the stress of looking after someone who may not remember who you are, can be devastating. Music and stress-reduction exercises can help devoted caregivers improve their own health as well. What better way than with music, to bring a smile to someone's face, and to lift their heart with joy? When music takes you to a place of inner peace, healing is not far behind.

## Resources for Healing

**Hum! Sing! Whistle!** One of the best things you can do to help your physical body get and stay well is to use the wonderful gift of your voice. We all have a built-in musical instrument which strengthens us and helps keep us whole. Use it! And please remember the power of playing any kind of musical instrument. The vibrations that you create when making music are powerful healers.

### Recommended Music:
*"Sound Healing,"* Dean Evenson & Soundings Ensemble
*"The Fairy Ring,"* Mike Rowland
*"Sound Body, Sound Mind,"* Andrew Weil

### Contemplation:
Some say that illness is a symptom of a disease of the soul. Something that is missing, or with which I have not dealt, is the root of the physical problems I suffer. Do I have something I should be dealing with? Do I have unresolved issues I should address?

### Affirmation:
I am strong, and healthy, and happy. All things, past and present, which have made it possible for me to become ill are resolved, and I release all pain and trauma. I am whole.

(There is a wonderful author named Louise Hay who has a series of books with affirmations for particular illnesses. We highly recommend that you read some of her work for additional recommendations.)

### Mantra:
Whole and healthy is my way.

# The Power of Music and Love

(a true story of the power of love in a song)

Karen had a three year old son, Michael, when she found she was pregnant with a baby girl. To encourage Michael's acceptance of the new baby, and to make him feel important, Karen encouraged the toddler to sing to his new sister. Every day, he sang to his baby sister as she rested in Mommy's tummy.

The pregnancy progressed normally, but when the baby was born, complications arose, and the baby had to be placed in a neonatal intensive care unit. The baby's condition worsened daily, and it seemed that she would not survive.

During his sister's illness, little Michael begged his mom to let him see his baby sister. He wanted to sing to her. Despite dire warnings from hospital staff, Karen brought her son to see the baby. She feared it would be the only time he would ever see her, and she was determined to let him sing to her.

Little Michael approached his baby sister, gazing at her for a moment. Then he began to sing the song he had been singing to her for the whole of her life:

*"You are my sunshine, my only sunshine,*

*you make me happy, when skies are gray... "*

Almost at once, the baby girl responded. Her pulse rate calmed down and became steady.

*"You never know, dear, how much I love you,*

*Please don't take my sunshine away."*

The baby's ragged, strained breathing became smooth and calm. "Keep on singing, sweetheart," Karen encouraged Michael.

*"The other night, dear, as I lay sleeping,*

*I dreamed I held you in my arms... "*

This tiny baby girl began to relax. Michael kept singing, Karen beamed, and the hospital staff stood amazed, as the baby fell into a peaceful sleep. The very next day, the baby girl was well enough to go home, to finally be with her big brother, Michael.

(*"You Are my Sunshine"* by Jimmie Davis and Charles Mitchell) ♪

*In the mother,*
*when the first trace of life*
*begins to stir,*
*music is the nurse of the soul.*
*It murmers in the ear*
*and the child sleeps.*
*The tones are the companions*
*of his dreams.*
*They are the world in which*
*he lives.*

*Antoine Bettina*

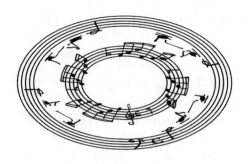

# FOUR

# Music and Emotion

*"Music can do two things. It can build
bridges and make people understand each
other and their differences.
Or it can dig the ditch and make the
problem bigger.
Rap is making the problem bigger."*

*Phil Collins*

A fourteen year old girl with green hair, purple lipstick, and a ring through her upper lip stood in front of us as we played. She listened, entranced, as the pure notes of a simple tune emanated from Kate's harp and Richard's acoustic guitar. No synthesizers, no bass, no drums, no words. Just a melody. She remained motionless. We didn't know what she was thinking.

Then, suddenly, this woman-child began to cry. The tears ran freely down her cheeks, mingling with the purplish blush on her cheeks. When the piece was over, she came to us and took Kate's hand. "Thank you," she said. Then she hurried away, still sniffing back some tears as she returned to the clatter and confusion that is Las Vegas.

It is moments like this that keep us playing our music in even the most difficult environments. Every day we see intense reactions. This girl's tears were by no means unique. Such an emotional response to music has happened to most of us at one time or another.

What is it about music that causes us to react so emotionally to it? Why do so many people intuitively search out music when they feel unsettled or unwell, or when they are dying?

We've discussed the physical effects of frequencies bombarding our body. We've seen how tones and vibrations can help cure cancer and headaches. These are all scientifically calibrated, measurable effects of sound.

But music is, of course, much more than frequencies and tones arranged in a mathematically precise order creating melody, countermelody, and harmony. It is a powerful force, and it is the emotional effect that most of us recall when we think of the power of music.

Even the famous psychoanalyst, Carl Jung, recognized the immense power of music on the human psyche. He felt that music should be a part of every analysis, because it could reach down inside and touch the very core of the individual. The root of a person's problems could be reached with music when many other methods failed.

*"The noble minded man's music is mild and delicate,*
*keeps a uniform mood, enlivens and moves.*
*Such a man does not harbor pain or mourn in his heart;*
*violent and daring movements are foreign to him."*

*Confucius*

An interesting story demonstrating the power of music on emotion comes from ancient Greece. There was a young Sicilian man who was at what would be equivalent to one of our bars. A flutist was playing music in a mode called Phrygian, definitely not a relaxing, melodic kind of music. As this young Sicilian sat listening to the music, he became more and more enraged. He believed that his lover had been having an affair and he was determined to go to her house and set it on fire. The longer the music played, the angrier this young man became.

Finally, the famous mathematician Pythagoras, who was also at the bar, realized what was happening and ordered the musician to stop playing that music. The flute player switched his music to a different mode and played a beautiful, soothing, melodic piece. Immediately the young Sicilian became calm and returned to his home completely passive.

## Inspiring Love or Fear

How many movies have you seen where the hero has to destroy the juke box or leave the room when a particular song is playing? The music evokes painful memories, inspiring him to violence, or to drink too heavily. Or, the opposite occurs. Someone puts a quarter in the machine, a beautiful tune begins to play, and a couple spy each other across the room. Their eyes meet, they fall into each other's arms and dance their way to romance.

Have you ever noticed the important role music plays when you have a new love interest in your life? Many of us remember the song that was playing when we first met, or the first tune to which we danced. Most couples have a song they consider theirs, and hearing it inspires warm memories for years to come.

Held closely to their mother's bosom, many babies are lulled to sleep by the mellow, lingering notes of *Rock a Bye Baby"* or *"Brahms Lullaby."* With music, a mother guides her intense love to her child during this bedtime ritual, inspiring feelings of safety and warmth. For a newborn, or even a baby in utero, music is the language of love. And years or decades later, the sound of a beloved lullaby can actually slow the heartrate and lower the blood pressure of senior citizens who heard those tunes as infants.

This emotional response is not limited to humans. Animals are affected by it as well. There was a veterinarian in Los Angeles during the 1970s who used beautiful violin music to calm his canine and feline patients. The animals were in such a state of contentment they evidently did not want to leave. Pet owners were amazed, and the veterinarian's business prospered. This doctor wanted his special four-footed patients to know that he loved each and every one of them, and to him, there was no better way than to play music that conveyed that emotion.

If music is a powerful emotional trigger for individuals, it follows that the emotions triggered by music can effect not only individuals and societies, but the course of history. Emotions inspired by music travel throughout Earth and the universe.

---

*"Music soothes us, stirs us up;*
*it puts noble feelings in us;*
*it melts us to tears, we know not how."*

Charles Kingsley

---

It becomes very important, then, to seriously consider what we're sending out with our music. There are really only two emotions—love and fear. All other emotional responses emanate from them. So does the music we make or listen to inspire love or fear?

If it's true that thought *creates* (and we believe that it does), then the thoughts conjured up by the emotional response to music can also create. And if the emotion and thoughts are negative or hateful, then it follows that destruction is a natural consequence.

*"Some people have a great sense of moral responsibility; unfortunately, it's backed up with a poor sense of musical taste. Other people have great musical ability, and very little sense of moral responsibility."*

*Eric Clapton*

So much of music today is full of hate and desire for revenge. These attributes come from the emotion of fear, which sends out more vibrations of fear. Anger flows from the fear, wreaking havoc and creating disease. Think of the impact harsh tones, grating effects, and foul vocals have on children. A child exposed to this kind of music on a constant basis will have a very different outlook on life than the child raised with Brahms and Bach.

Consider the pop musical changes in our society just since the 1950s and 1960s. Then, Elvis sang *"Love Me Tender"* and the Beatles cried *"She Loves You."* Harmony and strong melodies defined the music, and the lyrics centered around innocent love and relationships. People left their doors open and they certainly didn't worry that their child would be shot at school.

In the years since, especially the last twenty years, it's as if pop music has moved from a "G" to an "R" rating. You can hear it. Much of the music bought by young adults has become harsher and less melodic. The explicit lyrics are graphic; depicting sex, racial hatred, violence against women and authority figures, and rebellion against all that holds the society together. Believe it or not, many recordings today are actually sold with warning stickers on them. The point of the music is not to bring together the society, but to alienate its members and divide it into subcultures.

Is it any wonder, then, that children are killing children, adult children are abusing their elderly parents, and total strangers shoot someone who accidentally cuts them off in traffic? A full generation of people have now been exposed to this *angry* music. Their definition of the world comes from this dictionary of sound—this music filled with anarchy.

> "If I speak in the tongues of men and angels,
> but have not love,
> I am a noisy gong or a clanging cymbal."
>
> St. John the Apostle

So what do we do? This is a free country. We can't stop the creation of this music. We can't pass laws to make it go away. Even if we tried, it would just go underground and become an even more desirable forbidden fruit to those who feel they're being denied something. The makers and sellers of this music would succeed. The fear they inspire would manifest in paranoia and useless posturing by politicians and sociologists and media watchdogs. The government, in all its wisdom, could try to further regulate the content of recordings, movies and video games, but it wouldn't help. It would only inspire more of the same.

*Know at the very essence of your Being,*
*that the way of transforming*
*your life and that of those around you, is*
*through Love.*

*Anonymous*

Music created in the spirit of love sends positive energy into the universe and the people in it. Peace, hope, and joy all stem from the emotion of love. We counteract fear, hate, and paranoia by sending these positive, loving vibrations out to all within its reach. We expose society's members—especially the younger people who are wracked by fear—to music of beauty and grace that uplifts and enlightens.

Western society has been exposed to lower, dark forms of music for so long, it is gradually slipping into the Darkness. To bring it to the Light, we have to consciously change the soundtrack of this society and that of the planet.

Let's bring the pure tones of flutes, violins, chants, harps, and Native American drums to the masses. If parents were to play this kind of music to their unborn children and infants, if teachers played it in classrooms, and mall managers played it over the sound system—what a difference they could make. If all of us who yearn to make beautiful, loving music picked up and played an instrument or started to sing, think of the energy flowing into the universe! How wonderful it would be if an entire generation heard more music of love than music of fear.

So often we feel afraid because we feel alone and vulnerable in a frightening world. But when we sit quietly, listening to the music of angels, we remember that we are surrounded by love and we can open our hearts to the miracles of everyday life. If we can spread the emotion of love through music, then each of us will find health and inner peace more easily attained.

*Music should go right through you,*
*leave some of itself inside you,*
*and take some of you with it*
*when it leaves.*

Henry Threadgill

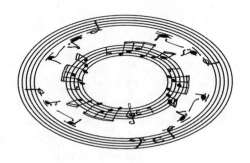

**FIVE**

# Music for Stress Reduction

*"We must do our business faithfully,*
*without trouble or disquiet,*
*recalling our mind to God mildly,*
*and with tranquillity,*
*as often as we find it wandering from Him."*

*Brother Lawerence,*
*"The Practice and Presence of God"*

We hate to be cliché and cash in on the disease of the century, but, we can't send you on a journey to inner peace if you're stressed out and running from morning till night. Stress is the number one problem most people have to deal with. Stress from money problems, work problems, family concerns, health, even the commute to work... the list is endless. When we perform our concerts or do our healing music workshops, the most common ailment people talk to us about is stress.

People turn to alcohol, drugs, promiscuous sex, all in a misguided effort to reduce what they perceive as stress. At the other end of the spectrum, millions, maybe billions, of dollars are spent each year on stress reduction. Psychotherapy, massage, yoga classes, meditation classes, retreats—these are just a few examples of the way people try to relax.

But on the way back from their yoga class, vacation, or retreat, they have to contend with gridlock, road rage, and carbon monoxide fumes. When they get home, the kids are coming at them from all directions, somebody wants dinner, and the TV is blaring out the latest terrible news. They go back to work the next day, where a pile of work awaits them, the phone doesn't stop ringing, and they have to learn a new computer program or risk getting downsized. It's very difficult in modern life to stay connected to that part of yourself which gives you joy and peace. It's hard to live with love in your heart when all you can really think about is getting away.

Stress destroys the peace within. Stress robs the mind's ability to focus on the things in life that bring pleasure and contentment. We've all experienced varying levels of stress in our lives, some more than others, and when stress gets out of control, dangerous degrees of subtle emotional and physical change begin to take place. This is where the right kind of music can bring relief.

If an individual is stressed out, listening to a screeching heavy metal tune from Metallica may make matters worse. Then again, listening repeatedly to "It's a Small, Small World" may drive him completely off the deep end. The type of music required for stress reduction and elimination is the type that allows your mind to wander peacefully. The music is a conduit for your imagination, permitting you to remove yourself from the sources of your stress.

## A Place of Peace

Try this yourself right now with "*Millennium*," the CD enclosed in this book. Listen to the first cut. Close your eyes, breathe deeply, and let your mind wander through a tranquil valley of peace. Think about the color of the sky, the beauty of the butterflies, the heat of the sun. Let your imagination soar. Just wander. Keep looking around at this place you've created. Remember its details.

While the music continues to play, imagine the stored up blackness of stress oozing completely out of your body. Imagine all that stress flowing away, leaving you completely. Your body will begin to unwind and feel physically relaxed.

As you relax, you will find thoughts of people and events that cause you stress coming into your mind. As each nagging worry, unpleasant thought, or remembered task comes to you, consciously acknowledge it, then say, "I'm relaxing right now. Let it be for now. I'll deal with you later." They will flit back out of your mind. They can wait. Every time they come back, say again, "Go away." Replace those thoughts with the picture of this peaceful place in which you are resting.

Feel the heavy weight of anxiety, stress and peer pressure give way to the light, airy feeling of finding a personal sanctuary that you will be able to return to time and time again. In 15 minutes you will emerge refreshed, rejuvenated, and so much happier.

## Family Time

Kids can have an incredible amount of pent up stress. Remember peer pressure, exams, and worrying about being the last one picked for the baseball team? Now, imagine what it must be like to be searched for weapons everyday. What's it like being around students who are selling speed, cocaine, and other drugs at even the most prestigious schools? It's very different being a kid today.

Stress manifests itself in temper tantrums, revolt, trouble at school, withdrawal, physical ailments and even suicide. It can affect a child's overall attitude to everything in life, including you, and accelerate the gap that often grows between a parent and a young adult.

Parents don't know what to do about it. They take their child to a doctor, who, because it's easier than dealing with the underlying sources of stress, diagnoses the disease of the decade, Attention Deficit Disorder, and starts the youngster on a drug. We know that a lot of the kids who are given drugs to stay focused or calm down might do much better if their parents or other caregivers shared a little music therapy with them.

Ask your son or daughter to join you on the sofa and close your eyes. Many people, especially children, find it difficult to really close their eyes, so a simple blindfold works well. Breathe deeply. Relax.

Gently guide your child to wander in his imagination to a place that is beautiful and green. (Green is an important color for stress relief.) There are lots of trees, and a stream running through a glade. You know your child, so you can help guide him to a place you may have visited on a family vacation or a place that looks like a picture in a favorite book. Help guide his imagination to that wonderful, peaceful place.

Then, tell him to imagine all the things that bother him falling into the stream. Or maybe he can throw them into the stream. They will be carried away and he can relax.

This is a very simple exercise for both of you, and is a wonderful way for you to spend valuable, quality time together.

## Active Stress Reduction

Sometimes it takes a little more to relax. You may run, work out at a gym, go dancing, maybe even box. All are excellent ways to tire the body physically and release pent-up physical tension.

It's absolutely true that you can eliminate stress and feel better emotionally if you feel good physically. Thus, whichever form of exercise you enjoy, do it regularly. And do it to music. Music helps you keep a rhythm to the workout, and helps you focus on the movements of your body.

Note: If you are going to do an aerobic workout to music, don't play it loudly in your headphones. Too much volume in the headphones can seriously damage your hearing because blood is being pumped to the lungs and limbs, away from the delicate tissues in the ears. They are sensitive to vibrations at this time.

## Take Time for Yourself

Kate was in a medical office recently, and on the wall was a poster that proclaimed "All I really need to know in Life, I learned in Kindergarten." Actually, it was the perfect recipe for life, and we'll paraphrase, since we don't remember it all.

*"Share your toys, pick up after yourself, don't be a bully, don't jump in line, cry if you want to, and always have a nap in the afternoon."*

We agree with all of these admonitions, especially the one to take a nap. When you were doing the listening exercise earlier in this chapter, we'll bet you started feeling drowsy. You may even have drifted off to sleep. That's good. One of the things we highly recommend for stress reduction is napping. Especially if you can fall asleep listening to some meditative, soothing music. Most importantly, let the music continue to play while you're sleeping.

Einstein and Edison, two of the most prolific and inventive thinkers of our time, often took naps. If they had used the language of today, they may have called them "power naps," because they were able to come up with the most incredible ideas after napping.

Most of us don't have the option of taking a nap in our office or at the factory, but nothing says we can't have one when we get home from work. Unless you have a hungry child or a pet that needs walking, nothing is so pressing that you can't take a break before you prepare dinner. Put *"Millennium"* in the CD player, close your eyes, and let it take you to a quiet, restful place. When you awaken, you will have a more enjoyable evening, and will feel much more peaceful.

Teachers should use gentle, soothing music to calm preschoolers and kindergarten students before their naps. The kids settle down much more quickly if they have soothing music than if they are just plunked down on their mats and told to "Be quiet and go to sleep!" Use that technique with your small children at home. The great side effect is that it will calm you, too.

Another incredible way to deal with stress is to take a music break every day, or several times in a day. Whether you're at home dealing with a fussy two year old, at work dealing with a cantankerous boss, or on the road in heavy traffic, music is a very positive antidote to stress.

If possible, when your workday gets rough, take a few minutes away from things and just sit quietly, listening to music like that which is included with this book. It will slow down your heartrate, lower your blood pressure, and generally make you feel more peaceful. You will be able to think better and deal with difficulties more easily.

We give this advice to people in our workshops, and often get responses like, "I'm so stressed! How can I relax when I worry that the time I take relaxing is taking away from things I'm supposed to be doing? If I don't get these things done, I'm even more stressed!" That is indeed a conundrum, but think about the state of your life. If you can't take time to attend to your own emotional and spiritual needs, how are you ever going to have the strength to attend to all of the other things in your life?

And even if you do take the time and make the effort to reduce the stress in your life, you can't force yourself to be at peace. It's like forcing yourself to be happy. It's impossible. All you can really do is be in the present, in the now. If you keep that in mind, as you listen to music, as you go about your daily chores, you will feel much more peaceful.

> *"We are like fish swimming in a sea of peace, refusing to acknowledge it as we breathe its very essence. The time will come when we will know what we breathe..."*
>
> *Alan Harris*

Everything that we recommend to you is aimed at creating a place of peace within. If something doesn't work for you, that's all right. But it's also okay to try, to take the time to do it. Stress is not compatible with inner peace. You're worth the effort it takes to reduce stress, so that you can be healthier and happier through any challenges this human experience hands you.

*Sing and dance together and be joyous,*
*but let each one of you be alone,*
*even as the strings of the lute are alone*
*though they quiver with the same music.*

*Kahlil Gibran*

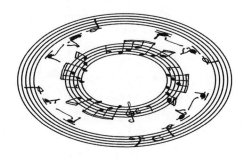

# SIX

# Healing Sadness and Depression

*"If we can love the stars*
*without knowing the vastness of the sky,*
*We can believe in miracles.*
*If we can believe in rainbows after the darkest storm,*
*We can believe in hope.*
*Somewhere beyond the clouds, behind the rain,*
*There are a thousand rainbows.*
*One is finding its way to you."*

*Anonymous, from the Internet, 1999*

At one time or another, most of us have suffered from the blues. Business or family pressures, periods of time away from loved ones, or even returning to work after an especially enjoyable vacation can make us feel out of sorts and kind of sad. Usually it lasts a few hours or days at most, and a funny movie or a walk in a favorite spot is all we need to shake the mood.

It's okay to have these down periods, because we all need the time and headspace to coddle ourselves a bit. We need to re-evaluate things in our life, and sometimes we can only do that if we're in a reflective, maybe even sad state of mind.

But when these episodes become increasingly frequent, of longer duration, and finally all-consuming, that is depression. Loneliness, isolation, despair, and hopelessness take over. Getting out of bed in the morning becomes a major achievement. For these unfortunate souls, the ideal of having inner peace may seem as unattainable as a lottery jackpot.

Depression doesn't show up on cat scans, x-rays, and blood tests. Those who are close to someone suffering from it have difficulty understanding that exhortations and threats cannot force their loved one to snap out of it. And while those suffering from depression often feel that it is their own personal hell, the fact is that those closest to them are also suffering.

There are many medications that supposedly alleviate depression. While these drugs may in fact control the symptoms, they cannot cure the illness. The cause must be searched out and eradicated. Regression and psychotherapy, hypnosis and even re-birthing sessions are all excellent ways of dealing with the issues that contributed to the depression. But a very useful, easily accessible healing tool is usually ignored.

That tool, of course, is the secret power of music. Whether you suffer occasional bouts of the blues or reside constantly in the depths of depression, music can have a powerful effect on your mental health. When the right kinds of music are combined with guided imagery and/or meditation, the effects on even severely depressed people can seem miraculous.

*Music is like a spiritual vitamin supplementing the soul with strength, certainty, and hopefulness.*

We've already talked about the effects that certain frequencies, tones, and vibrations have on the physical body. We've also considered our own emotional responses to various styles and genres of music. Now, we can use this knowledge of the power of music to dispel sadness and depression and claim the joy that is rightfully ours.

If someone were to ask you, "What's wrong? Why are you so sad?" What would you say? Do you feel you are too fat or too skinny, not attractive, or smart enough? Don't make enough money, have enough friends, or someone who loves you? When you consider all the things that we think are wrong with our lives, it's a wonder any of us gets through this life with a smile. We are just not happy with ourselves.

We're waiting for that promotion, to lose weight, to get a new car, to have a baby... then we'll be happy. But of course, even when we get any or all of those things, there's no guarantee they'll make us happy. All we've achieved is a great job, a perfect body, a fast car, a baby. What happens when you realize that there is nothing else to which you can aspire?

The worst thing that could happen is to realize that there is no hope of finding happiness, because there is nothing left to conquer or acquire. There is nothing out there that gives you joy. So what do you do? You have to remember: joy and happiness are within, living right alongside peace. You just have to greet and embrace them. You must become aware that you already possess all that you need to be genuinely happy.

Each one of us is a very powerful, spiritual being. We are all sparks from the same Light that is the Creator. If we can stay in touch with the powerful creator that is inside, we can recognize that we create our own happiness. We don't have to depend upon anything or anyone else for joy.

But in order to listen to the inner, creative you, you must first learn to hear your inner self over all of the clatter that surrounds our modern life.

## Listen

Go to the quietest space you can find, and just sit for five minutes or so. Sit quietly. Listen. At first you may think you hear nothing, but it will come. Listen to the hum of an air conditioner, the chirping of a bird, the wind rustling through the trees, or the buzz of electricity in high tension wires. Listen to each of these sounds individually. Focus on them, one at a time. You will begin to feel them deep inside; they will develop a rhythm to you.

If you sit long and quietly enough, you will begin to hear your own body. You may even want to cover your ears so that you can really focus on your own internal sounds. You will hear (maybe for the first time) your own breathing. Listen to the beating of your own heart. Regulate your breathing. Change its rhythm. Listen.

*Train your heart to listen.*

Now, use this newfound skill by listening to a piece of music. *"Millennium"* is great because the pure tones arranged in simple melodies allow your mind to focus, and you can practice conscious hearing. Listen to the music with the same attentiveness you've just given to the silence and your own body. Let it transport you to a place within yourself where you may remember events and people which have caused you sadness or disappointment. If these things are making you depressed, it may be because you've made a judgment about their value to you.

Don't let judgments prevent you from seeing the good that lies beyond experiences. Release your judgments, and enjoy. If you're honest with yourself, you'll probably see that there is no reason to feel bad about these things or people. This may give you an immense feeling of relief, which may cause you to cry.

That's a good thing, because crying releases pent up emotions, and allows negative energy to flow from the body. You then need to replace that negative energy with positive thoughts and feelings, expressed in affirmations such as the following:

*I am the master of my own destiny. I decide now that I am happy and content.*

*I am beautiful, powerful, and creative. I can do anything.*

*I am in the best place I can be, right now.*

Continue listening to the music for awhile. Create your own affirmations that confirm what you know in your mind, and in your heart—that you are the master of your own happiness.

Go a step further. Imagine yourself in a place of beauty, a place of peace. Picture the most beautiful place you can be, and be there.

Feel joy and peace flooding over you, becoming part of you. Use the music to take your self to that place now, and every time you begin to feel unhappy. Remember always that you created that beautiful place and those positive feelings, and they are yours whenever you want them.

## Forgive and Be Forgiven

While you're in this place of peace created by you and the music, you may begin to think of other things that are making you feel bad. Is there someone who you feel has hurt you? Are you harboring resentment toward that person? Unresolved issues like this have a way of festering into depression and other emotional problems, and you should take this opportunity to get rid of them.

You may not be able to talk directly to those individuals, but you can imagine that you're meeting them to clear the air. Allow yourself to be drawn into the music again, into your peaceful place, and as you are, imagine that these individuals are there with you, standing in front of you. They are smiling, as are you. Notice what they are wearing, how they look. Really look at them, into their eyes. Address each of them individually, saying:

> *"I forgive you, completely, and freely. I set you free, and let you go to that which is the best for you. All is cleared up between us, now and forever. I let you go to your own peace."*

Now consider the people that you may have hurt. That includes yourself. Have you done something which has caused grief or pain to someone else? They may not even be aware of it, but you are. You hold it inside you. Now is the time to clear the air. Imagine again, that you are in your peaceful, safe place, and they are there. Hear them telling you that you are forgiven. Everything is cleared up between you, and you can go to your own peace. You will be astonished at how much happier you feel once you've learned to give and accept forgiveness.

## Create Your Joy

We've said this many times in this book, and we'll say it again, because it is *so* important. To truly see your self, recognize your worth, and feel at peace, nothing is as potent as creating. Especially if you are creating music. With your voice, or with an instrument, this manifested act of creation will give you joy.

A part of your soul is stimulated when you make music. It is an honest, uncensored purging of the Self. Release your pent up fears, anxieties, sadness, by singing. Sing the blues, if you want. Make up a song explaining why you have the blues. Beat on a drum, play a flute. Strum a guitar. Make your own kind of music.

You've cleared the air. You've addressed long-standing issues. You've realized your power as a creator. You can push sadness and feelings of self-loathing away, and open your heart. You can see and enjoy the abundance that you have been given and that you have created yourself. In this glorious state of acceptance and joy, depression just cannot prevail, and inner peace and healing will be yours.

♪ *This existence of ours is as transient*
*as autumn clouds.*
*To watch the birth and death of being*
*is like looking at the movements of a dance.*
*A lifetime is like a flash of lightning in the sky,*
*rushing by, like a torrent*
*down a steep mountain.*

*The Buddha* ♪

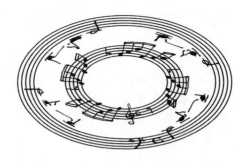

## SEVEN

# To Everything There is a Season

*"To everything there is a season,*
*And a time for every purpose under heaven...*
*A time to be born, a time to die,*
*A time to kill, a time to heal;*
*A time to mourn and a time to dance..."*

*The Book of Ecclesiastes, Ch. 3*

While we were writing this book in the summer of 1999, our beautiful 10-year-old wolf dog, Timber, was killed while on a morning walk with Kate. A negligent driver, speeding on the wrong side of the road, grazed Kate, then struck our "little girl."

For the first time in our married life together, we were faced with a terrible event over which we had no control. We could do nothing to fix it. No amount of work, tears, ranting, prayer—not even music—could bring her back.

Timber was a perfect little spirit radiating love wherever she went. She was the closest we had to a child, and she was our inspiration. The love she gave us was sent on through our music to everyone around us. What were we to do without our guiding light? From where would our inspiration come? Timber's passing changed us forever, and forced us to face one human emotion that everyone must face sooner or later. Grief.

In fact, just a week after Timber was killed, John F. Kennedy Jr. and his family died in a plane crash. We experienced grief anew; this time as empathetic standers-by, mourning with a nation for the loss of more bright lights. It compounded yet again with shootings in a church in Texas, a devastating earthquake in Turkey, killer floods in North Carolina, and another shooting at a preschool in California. It seemed that everywhere, wonderful souls were being taken, and families were left to grieve.

With these events coming so close together, we were able to speak to many people about grief. People who normally would not have talked with us about their losses, shared them, and we worked together to ease our collective pain. We grieved not only for the lives that were lost, but also for the opportunity, hope, and vitality that was destroyed when they died.

It made us realize that grief is not only for a lost loved one; it is also for lost opportunities. It is for the loss of innocence, for the loss of hope and freedom. We all have unfinished business, unspoken words, lost moments, and unresolved issues. We come to realize that we may never be able to accomplish certain things, and we grieve for time that is lost.

As spiritual beings going through this human existence, grief is one of the most difficult things with which we all must deal sooner or later. It doesn't matter how much consolation others try to give you, or how many other people are going through the same thing, or how many words and cards and flowers come to comfort you; there is just no easy way out of grief.

We were forced by the events of the summer of 1999 to pay attention to grief. While we wish our attention had been brought here some other way, we embrace this opportunity to share now, how music helped us and others work through grief, and to find peace and healing within ourselves.

---

*"So ending flows to beginning*
*Like the cry of a swan*
*We are in a sickroom*
*But the night belongs to the angels"*

*Nelly Sachs*

---

Denial, anger, guilt, depression, acceptance, and resolution. These are the stages of grief. You may go through them in that order, or you may not. But most likely, you will go through them all. You need to. You must confront all of the stages of grief, so that the residue of these powerful emotions do not harm you physically or spiritually.

# Anger

Anger threatened to destroy us when Timber was killed. From anger sprung the desire for revenge, the desire to destroy the person who had caused our despair. We wanted that negligent teenage driver to hurt as much as we did. We wanted her to suffer pain like Timber had.

Forgiving wasn't even a consideration, as far as we were concerned. There was no way to get any satisfaction out of anyone. For the first time, we understood how parents of a child killed by a drunk driver or survivors of a school shooting or a terrorist bombing could be so consumed with the desire for revenge that nothing else mattered in their lives. Hating the "bad guy" gives us something upon which to focus our pain.

Oftentimes, though, there really isn't anyone with whom you can be angry. When you lose someone to old age or a heart attack, who takes the brunt of your anger? Someone has to take the blame, so you become angry at the medical system, or your loved one for abandoning you, or at just anyone or anything that crosses your path.

This is a very difficult stage to get through, because it's easier to be mad than to be sad. It doesn't hurt as much to rant and rave and plot revenge as it does to just feel sadness and despair. How do you pass through this destructive, irrational stage?

It is far from easy. But there is help. Calming, peaceful music is absolutely invaluable during this stage. Allow yourself to be soothed by gentle, wandering music. This is not the time to listen to angry, complicated music. Your body needs to receive frequencies that will slow it down; your emotions need to be soothed. You need to confront the anger and dismiss it—gently.

To help with that, we developed the following meditation. Using some of the ideas from the *Tibetan Book of Living and Dying* (which we highly recommend), we devised this process.

You must physically relax. Play *"Millennium,"* breathe deeply, relax all the muscles in your body, then, read these words, over and over, until you understand them:

> *I am angry right now—at the world, at God, at myself. Even though I know that death is real, and that every atom, every person, every thing dies, that there is no escaping Death, I want to blame everyone and everything for this tragedy. I believe that every death has some purpose. It's not easy to see that purpose right now, but I know that there is a plan of which I am a part. I do not want my anger to interfere with the peaceful transition of my loved one's soul, and so I am releasing the anger. I am releasing their soul to the All That Is, and to the Light and Life that is beyond this earthly plane.*

You won't instantly feel better (nothing is instant in this process of grieving), but keep remembering those words. Reflect upon them often. They will ring true to you eventually; especially if, at the same time, you listen calmly to music that inspires peace. Once you have truly addressed your anger, you can release it and learn to accept what has happened.

## Guilt

"What if I had taken another street? What if I'd booked an earlier flight? Why didn't I kiss him before he walked out that door?" How many people think or say those very words when a loved one dies? They want to turn back the hands of time, change something they did, or something they said. They feel guilty about everything, perhaps even for the fact that they are living.

97

For Kate, guilt was all-consuming. "If I had stepped to the right instead of the left. If I had played with Timber on the lawn one more minute. If I had only moved faster."

Even if you really had nothing to do with why your loved one passed away, you may feel guilty—for not listening to a friend who was in pain, for not calling your Grandmother on her last birthday, for not saying you loved your spouse—the list is endless.

How many times have we heard of a child drowning in the family pool? Many times we hear of the parents breaking up after this kind of event. Guilt and blame destroy the relationship just when the parents need each other the most.

One gentleman we know, whose wife was killed in a car crash on a rainy afternoon, blames himself for letting her go out that day. He wonders if he could have put better tires on the car, maybe he could have made her wait until the rain stopped. For years, this man blamed himself for an accident over which he had no control. He drank to excess, took drugs, dropped out of society. His guilt very nearly destroyed him. It is only now, nearly twenty years later, that he has come to grips with the fact that he was not to blame. He has learned to forgive himself.

You must do the same. If you are feeling guilt over the loss of someone or something, you must forgive yourself. You must also forgive the one that left you.

## An Exercise in Forgiving

Put on some beautiful, soothing music, like *"Millennium,"* or any meditative, instrumental music. Breathe deeply, and close your eyes.

Now, imagine yourself in a beautiful place. Perhaps a garden, or by the ocean. You are standing in front of your dearly departed. They are whole, healthy, complete. Or, imagine that the opportunity you missed, or the chance you had, is in front of you. Embody that lost chance. Give it the form of a person.

Imagine yourself apologizing to your lost one. Hear yourself saying the words, "I'm so sorry. I feel that I made a mistake. I feel bad. Can you ever forgive me?"

Now, imagine that your loved one forgives you. Hear him or her say the words:

"I forgive you. You did nothing wrong. There is nothing to feel guilty about. I'm sorry that I had to leave you, and I would have stayed if it had been the right thing, but I had to move on. I love you."

Hear and accept these words. Listen to your loved one say them over and over again. Hear the words, feel the love. You must accept that guilt will not bring anyone or anything back. It will only destroy you. Allow yourself to be forgiven. Allow yourself to forgive the person who left you.

As you come out of this exercise, give yourself a hug. Don't just go on to the rest of your life right away. Remember the feeling of peace you just experienced. Hold onto it. You can pull it back to yourself whenever you need it. Use the music as often as you need to transport you to your loved one, and to remind you of forgiveness.

## A Chance to Grow

We've known many widows or widowers who, after losing their spouses, simply decide that there's no reason to go on. The fact that there is one less set of footsteps, one less place to set, is more than they can bear, and they allow depression to take over. Suddenly, their lives are empty. There is no real reason to even get up in the morning. Why clean an empty house?

During our lives, we are always striving to fill ourselves up with knowledge, excitement, or power. We fill our lives with caring for other people, with keeping company, with learning and growing.

Death stops us. Grief empties us. It forces us to closely examine the vessel that is our Self. In that way, grief is a very powerful and good thing, because how are we to grow spiritually if all we do is fill up our consciousness? Allow yourself to be still, and to feel the emptiness.

Every virtuoso knows that the pauses between notes is where the true art in music resides. It is true also in the art of being a complete human being. Only when you feel the emptiness can you really feel your soul. It is here, in this empty place, that music can be especially powerful.

Again, play the *"Millennium"* CD. Just listen to the music. As you listen, allow it to transport you outside of your body. Just sit back and look at you: who and what you truly are all by yourself. You have things, do things, create things—and you will remember those first—but who are you really?

What is it about your personality, your very being, that defines you? Does it have anything to do with the person for whom you are grieving? If you are grieving for lost opportunities, are you any less a person than you would have been if you had accomplished something that you did not?

What we're getting at here, is that you should take this opportunity that grief gives you, to really examine yourself. The vessel that is you feels empty now. Are you going to fill it back up the way it was, or are you going to be different? Embrace this opportunity to decide.

# Connecting Through Music

Now and throughout the ages, music has been a conduit for comfort. It can be your best friend. It has order, harmony, and purpose. It is re-assuring, especially music that comes to us during rituals such as funerals or memorials. Through music, there is an avenue for expression; an avenue that everyone can understand. By its very nature, music connects us together.

At funerals, music is chosen to exemplify the deceased, and to make the mourners connect with parts of themselves and their dearly departed. These rituals involving music are a great comfort to us, as are things like lighting candles, laying flowers, even wearing black. They allow common mourning, common expression. A chance to embrace, and be embraced. They allow us to express the emptiness that accompanies the loss of a loved one.

In civilizations throughout history, chanting and singing are an integral part of the grieving process. In medieval France, certain chants were prescribed for those who were ill, and a series of chants were used to accompany the dying in their passage to the beyond. Based on passages or themes in the bible, these chants were sung in praise of God, inspiring listeners and singers alike to feel a connection to the Holy Spirit. And at a time of great mourning, this connection to the Creator is paramount in dealing with grief.

This is true even if you are furious at the Creator for causing you this grief. Connecting to what you may consider the source of your pain may be necessary if you are to release the anger and blame.

Have you ever listened to Mozart's *Requiem Mass?* Mozart wrote this masterpiece just before he died. It is filled with all the magnificence of life and the finality of death. This piece pulls out of you emotions and feelings you may not have realized you had. Few compositions can help purge a griefstruck heart like this. It encourages raging grief, tentative hope, and, most comforting to us, reverence for the Almighty.

Like so much of the great music of all civilizations, this piece seems almost to transcend the physical in which we operate. If we truly listen, and absorb the effect of this music, we can feel the inspiration from which it came. It is like a window to the beyond, a connection to the dimensions we cannot see, but can feel through music.

And where are our departed loved ones, but beyond this dimension in which we live. Great music like this gives us a connection to those who have gone on before us, a connection we would never want to lose.

*"When involved in worldly things,*
*You never think of death's approach;*
*Quick it comes like thunder*
*Crashing round your head."*

*Milarepa*

## Acceptance

Finally, you will come to accept your grief. You will accept that your loved one is never coming back. You will learn that life does go on, and amazingly, you will find that there are things to be joyful about. You will be able to face the memories with joy instead of sorrow. You will be able to smile again.

Something as simple as a beautiful sunset or a butterfly will give you joy when you come out of the blackest part of grief. Embrace these small miracles. Listen to some happy music. Dance! Sing! Whistle! There is so much for which we can be thankful. When you discover all these wonders, even in the face of your pain, you will truly have found your peace within.

*Musical training is a more potent
instrument than any other,
because rhythm and harmony
find their way into the inward
places of the soul,
on which they mightily fasten,
imparting grace, and making
the soul of him who is rightly educated,
graceful.*

Plato

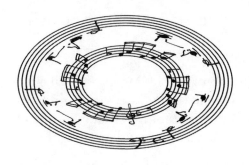

# EIGHT

# The Soundtrack
# of Our Lives

*"Stummin' my pain with his fingers,*
*Singin' my life with his words,... "*

from *"Killing me Softly with His Song"*
*Norman Gimble – Charles Fox*

From birth to death, our lives are accompanied by a soundtrack of music. Mostly, we take it for granted. It's just there—on the radio as we get dressed in the morning, through the headphones of our Walkman when we run or work out, in the vehicle next to us at the stoplight.

As infants, we are lulled to sleep by soft lullabies sung by our mothers. As we enter preschool and kindergarten, music is the fun way we are taught everything from our ABC's to what a cow says. Can you imagine learning the alphabet without the song? In grammar school, the sing-song memory aids for spelling and grammar go a long way toward helping us master the finer points of the English language. Remember "i" before "e" except after "c" and the "Months of the Year" song?

Come adolescence, music takes on a whole new meaning—it is the soundtrack of your teens. You will always remember the song that was playing when you met your first boyfriend or girlfriend, or when you broke up with someone you loved. At a wedding reception, the couple's special song is usually played as the first dance. The music played during the ceremony itself is also carefully chosen to set up exactly what you want to convey to your guests.

We recently watched an infomercial selling a CD, *"AM Gold of the Seventies."* What memories came to us as we watched television that night. Richard was a radio announcer during the '70s; spinning those songs every day. Kate was a teenager, dancing through adolescence and high school to the tunes of Tony Orlando and Dawn and K.C. and the Sunshine Band.

It was wonderful for us to grow up with relatively peaceful, easygoing music. Unfortunately, music has changed a lot in the last twenty-five years.

## Growing Up Today

Think about the effect that music has had on us over the last half a century. Just as you are what you eat, you are also what you listen to. There is a big difference between a person who listens to gangster rap and a person who listens to new age or classical music. There's a marked difference between the teenager who listens to anti-establishment punk rock and the teenager who listens to more innocent, happier, pop music.

We often bemoan the youth of today. Kids are shooting other kids at school and committing acts of violence in their homes and neighborhoods. We point to the music and say, "See?" But it's not that simple. There are as many kinds of music as there are kids.

Here, then, is the question. Does the music make the kid, or do the kids make the music? Probably a bit of both. So we need to get kids to reject the music that inspires aggression. How do we do that?

What would happen if young adults were exposed to music that provided pure, round tones that were peaceful and reflective? We can almost hear what you're thinking. "Just how are we supposed to get these kids to listen to that kind of music?" It's not so difficult, really.

Where do kids hang out? Fast food restaurants, malls, the movie theaters. It's very easy to change the music in those places. What if the melodic but hip music by Loreena McKennitt, Enya, or Secret Garden was playing? The kids might decide they like it. There's nothing not to like. If you're not aware of the music we're mentioning, run, don't walk, to your nearest music store and listen to these artists.

## The Sounds of School

What do you think it would be like if carefully programmed music was playing over the public address system as kids were coming in to school? Why not have *"Celtic Odyssey"* or *"Sons of Somerled"* playing? How wonderful it would be to start the day that way instead of with endless diatribes from principals extolling the necessity of being on time and remembering the basketball game that afternoon.

Can you imagine if all schools started and ended their day with music? In the interests of equal rights, freedom of religion, and other fashionable causes, prayer has been taken out of schools. We find that very sad because it leaves no time or place for young people to collect and prepare themselves mentally or spiritually for their day. What if they started their school day with music? Could anyone object to peaceful music? Or would that, too, be considered politically incorrect? We hope that no one would complain because there wasn't equal time for rap or punk rock.

If students were given the opportunity to sit quietly for ten minutes first thing in the morning, maybe in home room, and for ten minutes at the end of the day, listening to peaceful, pure toned music, we bet they would have a different attitude toward school, and life in general. They'd feel more positive and less stressed. In the back of the book, we've listed our favorite "cool" new age recordings. We know lots of young people who enjoy them. Try them on your students, your children, your grandchildren.

There are so many opportunities to utilize the calming power of music in our society. It's unfortunate that music so often generates the opposite effect.

## Radio and Television

There are over one hundred radio stations in the Los Angeles market. You can hear rap, rock, hip hop, pop, country, latino, and more talking than you care to hear. But not one single LA station programs ambient, acoustic, or peaceful new age music as their prime format.

Sure, in many markets, National Public Radio airs their Sunday night *"Hearts of Space"* program, and the odd hour of University Radio plays some healing music, but it's very hard to find. Only a few commercial radio stations around the country air a permanent format of acoustic, ambient, or new age music. Why aren't there more stations playing this music that the world needs right now? It seems that radio stations have a big responsibility. They have the power to make hits out of music that can inspire violence. Now they should use that power to make hits out of music that will calm the world down. How about someone building a music radio station that programs music just to reduce stress, anger, and depression? It's time for broadcasters and everyone else in business to recognize the power of the music they play, not just the commercials they air.

## Sound Saturation

It's not just the radio that hammers away at our consciousness anymore. Wherever you go, whatever time of day, you are bound to hear music or a television playing somewhere. In your car, in the doctor's office, at the grocery store, in the shopping mall, in the elevator, at the beach, in a restaurant. It's playing all the time.

The relentless stream of tones and sound can and does affect your mood. Your thoughts and your emotional feelings are being influenced continually, and you are probably not even aware of it. It's the *soundtrack of our lives.* And that's why we're showing you in this book how to be very conscious of the music you hear. For as much as music can bring you joy and peacefulness, so, too, can it create discordance in your self and disease in your body. Don't leave it to chance.

# Business

One evening recently, we were in a nice restaurant celebrating our anniversary. The food was good, but loud jazz music was playing over the sound system. In the corners of the bar adjacent to the restaurant were two television sets—one tuned to a basketball game, the other to an old movie. Still another kind of music was being piped into the bar. There was so much noise in that building, by the end of the meal we were nervous wrecks.

What surprised us, was that most people didn't even seem to notice the noise. They just talked louder—to each other or on their cell phones—to get over the noise. This just typifies how noisy our society is, and how people have adjusted to it.

Business and store owners, employees, and restaurant managers all have their own idea of what kind of music best suits their outlet. The trouble is, most don't have a clue about what kind of music or ambiance is required. When this happens they stand to annoy and irritate their customers and perhaps lose them for good—as the above-mentioned restaurant has lost us.

Ever notice how wonderful it feels to shop in stores like the Nature Conservancy or the Discovery Store? As soon as you enter these retail shops you feel refreshed. What is it? What makes it different from entering a toy store or a jean shop? It's the ambient music being played.

Enter these shops and you will hear the sounds of Native American flutes, oceans, tropical rain forests, wolf howls, and waterfalls. The music creates a cove of tranquillity and peacefulness amidst the hectic din generated from the rest of the shopping mall. Being in these stores makes you want to linger. You can hear yourself think. You feel calmer, more relaxed... ready to buy.

We just saw a report that a number of large businesses and corporations have begun to use therapeutic music in the workplace. They are allowing some employees to use Walkman stereos and personal headphones, while other businesses are consulting music therapists to establish a "tonally correct" workplace. These efforts are proving to be extremely beneficial to emotional job health, resulting in high morale, increased productivity, and less sick days. We hope the rest of Corporate America is not far behind.

## The Healing Environment

We've mentioned it before, but we feel very strongly that hospitals and doctors' offices—these places where we are sent to be healed—are among the worst offenders in the "noise pollution" problem.

Kate recently had to undergo therapy for an arm and hand injury. During each treatment, the beeping, bleeping, whooshing, and other sounds of a hospital surrounded her, while next door in the chemotherapy unit the annoying soundtrack of a very loud TV soap opera blared. It was very discomforting, and certainly did nothing to enhance the healing process.

There simply has to be a better way for hospitals to handle noise. What if all hospitals played calming music in all the wards—would there be a difference? Would people heal more quickly, would they feel more comfortable, more hopeful? Of course they would. And with all the talk of rising healthcare costs, prescription drug abuse, and other problems in the healthcare system, it seems to us that music is worth the investment.

There is no question that music eases pain and reduces stress. If people heal faster and require fewer drugs, the cost of treatment has to go down. Something to ponder when choosing a medical facility.

Choose the music you allow into your life as carefully as you plan a diet. Listen to it with recognition of its power. If you use it with awareness and respect, music will take you on a joyous journey to health and peace within.

*"Our sound environment is
vital to our survival and growth
in this plane of existence."*

Joel Andrews

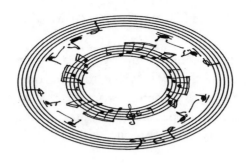

# NINE

# Create a Peaceful Environment

*"To be at peace is not to be in a place where there is no noise, trouble, or unpleasantries. To be at peace is to be calm in your heart in the midst of that which is not."*

*Kate Mucci*

The emotions conjured up by human interaction are very powerful. If they're allowed to enter our consciousness, then we have to recognize what it is that they are doing to us. The way we allow people or sounds, feelings or sights, to enter our consciousness determines how we feel about our own selves.

Once you become aware of the sonic and other influences that are always bombarding you, you will be able to turn anything negative into positive energy, and enhance the positive effects of all that is good.

It's not within the scope of this book to delve into all of the practices that allow you to deal with negative energy. There are many excellent books you can read and courses you can take to gain those skills. What we offer you here is a way to make your own personal space a place of peace and healing, and ways to use the power of music to help you get through this sometimes trying human experience.

---

*"And now it is an angel's song,*
*That makes the heavens be mute."*

*Anonymous*

---

## A Peaceful Space

Sound is one of the most pervasive influences in our lives. Many of us live near busy streets and freeways, airports, even railroad tracks. It's often difficult to sleep, and people living close to noisy places like that often feel stressed and jumpy. It's easy to say,

"Well, then, move!" but we all know it's just not that easy. So, we have to deal constructively with the noise that invades our space.

If it is possible to soundproof your environment, do so. Take at least one room, perhaps the bedroom, and do whatever you can to make it a peaceful place. If you can use soundproofing materials, do so. Hang cork panels on the walls. Put heavy draperies and/or double pane glass in the windows. Put weather stripping around the windows to block out sound leakage.

Make this room your place of peace and healing. Imagine the most peaceful place you can, and try to emulate that feeling in your room. Add some beautiful flowers or plants, maybe even a small fountain. Be sure you have a way of playing music in the room, or have a personal stereo with headphones.

## Special Things

If you like, add an altar. Fill that altar with things that have great meaning for you. Perhaps crystals, momentos, or photographs. A feather, a bird's nest, seashells, or candles. All of the things that give you peace... put them in a sacred space in this room.

If you decide to enhance your room with crystals, make sure that you use them properly. To create a place of peace, the Blue Lace Agate is very powerful, as it calms your mind and helps to relieve stress. Amethyst, aquamarine, malachite, and sapphire are also very strong "peace makers."

Be sure that your crystals are cleansed—that is, simply wash them under running water (preferably a stream or river), or let them soak in water and sea salt overnight. Then, bless them as you bless your room, and convey love as energy to them. Remember, just as sound and music are energy, your own emotions are energy. If you send positive thoughts and love to

117

objects in your space, that energy will be enhanced and brought back to you. As you meditate and listen to music, you will be able to tap into that energy.

# Color

Color is a very important thing to consider in your environment as well. Remember that what we see as different colors are really no more than different portions of the light spectrum. It is various wavelengths of light. Light is energy, just like sound, and the energy from the colors with which you are surrounded also has an enormous impact on your sense of well being.

You know which colors make you feel peaceful, and which do not. If you are creating a place of peace and healing, then you must make sure that the colors in that space don't invoke other kinds of emotions in you.

Green is a powerful healing color. Brown is excellent for peace. Earthy colors generally create a sense of connecting to nature and finding peace there. Thus, the addition of warm wooden furniture and walls, plants, or artwork that depicts nature can go a long way in making your space more peaceful.

## Your Work Environment

The time you spend at work is often greater than the time that you actually get to enjoy your home. If you have an office or workspace that you can decorate, do so. Make it into a peaceful, comfortable space. If at all possible, have music playing. Obviously, you don't want to disturb co-workers, but it's a proven fact that certain types of music can increase productivity and job satisfaction. If you are more comfortable at your job, you will be healthier and happier.

## Sound Breaks

*Do not forget to pause when the distractions and pressures of daily life deplete your energy. A sound break gives you time to dream, to contemplate, to think. You will see more clearly what works in your life, in your job, and how you can change things to make them better.*

Sound breaks are wonderful. Many of us have periods in our day where our brains just want to shut down. For many people, it's mid-afternoon, that period after lunch when your brain would much rather be sleeping and letting all the oxygen go to your stomach for digestion. This is the time for a sound break. Stop working, and listen consciously to music that will invigorate you and increase your creativity. Don't just put it on in the background—stop and really listen to a favorite selection. Five minutes twice per hour during that difficult time in your day will be time well spent.

If you have a stressful job, music like *"Millennium"* is excellent for making work a calmer place. There are CDs on the market which are especially compiled for mental or creative work. A lot of Mozart's music has been categorized for specific situations and needs. Go to your local music store and explore the wonderful variety of music available.

If you work in a factory or other place where noise is a problem, make sure you get away from the noise whenever you can. If it won't affect your safety, wear earplugs. During your lunchbreaks, don't go into the noisy cafeteria if you can avoid it. Take your lunch outside, under a tree. Do a few deep breathing exercises, clear your mind and your heart. Listen to the silence, if you can. If even the outside is noisy, take your personal stereo and headphones with you, and listen to calming music. A break from the sensory overload of the job will definitely help you through the day.

## Simplify

There's no doubt that life is too complicated. Scale down. You don't win the game of life just because you have the most toys. In fact, our experience, and that of everyone we know, is that the more we have, the more we want, and the harder we have to work to hold onto it. That isn't what life is about. It certainly won't make you any healthier or help you sleep better at night.

Just before writing this book, we decided to change our life drastically. Instead of having a six-day-a-week job entertaining in a bustling city, we're on the road, teaching our *"Healing with Music"* workshops, playing in hospitals and hospices, and performing our *"Magical Music"* concerts in small towns across the country.

We simplified. Everything we need to live and work is right here with us, in a beautiful motorhome. We got rid of our apartment in Las Vegas, sold all our furniture, and are having the time of our lives. We're like turtles. No art collection, no fine china, no antiques, no mortgage, and a much reduced collection of electronic gadgets.

During our travels we've met many people like us. Everyone from fed-up doctors and ex-military types, to artists and disillusioned corporate executives have simplified their lives, condensing their possessions to a lifestyle on wheels. They are truly some of the happiest, most content people we've ever known.

Of course this is not everyone's idea of an ideal lifestyle. Not for one moment would we suggest that anyone give up their lifestyle for ours. But it can't hurt to scale down, to simplify your life. Is it really that important to have a sixty-inch TV when your forty-inch set is working just fine? Do you really need the latest 750mhz Pentium 3 computer when your 333mhz Pentium 2 computer is working perfectly? Is your life on such a fast track that five more seconds of time to download an image off the net will make or break your day? Why?

Simplify. Enjoy that which you have. If you have things that do not give you joy—get rid of them. Maybe someone else will get joy out of them. If you aren't enjoying them, they are complicating your life. Go through your house and give away or sell anything you haven't touched in two years. It's a wonderful experience.

Analyze for a few days or weeks what it is that truly makes you feel good. Is it walking your dog or reading? Is it making a nice meal of fresh foods for your family? Is it taking afternoon naps? Visiting Grandma on the weekend? Our guess is that when you really think about it, the things that make you the happiest are the simplest. Make those your focus, and you will experience a huge leap in your own sense of inner peace.

Nobody needs a lot of *stuff* to be happy. Simple is good. It relieves a lot of pressure, and gives you time to explore that which is truly important... the love of family and friends, nature, and your own sense of self. If you still feel the need to acquire, why not acquire music. Build the biggest music library in the neighborhood.

## Quality Time

When was the last time you sat with your family and played games? Was the TV on in the background? Probably. Have you ever sat with your family and just listened to music? Have you ever sat your young children on your knees, or curled up with your spouse, or your cat, and just listened to beautiful music? Please do it tonight.

Try this... *turn off the TV for a week and put on some music.* How about some popular classical music or one of the hot, new Celtic artists? Try something without lyrics if possible, that will allow you to converse with your family. Light a candle and really listen to the music.

If you have teenagers, this is a great time to ask them to share their music with you. And then share your music with them. This is not a time to critique... it is a time to experience and enjoy music for its own merits, and to enjoy the company of your family.

Discover the joy of just being, because life is a gift. If you've ever been very ill, or lost someone dear to you, you know how precious life is. Cherish it.

Keep the music in your peaceful place pure and simple. Peaceful, instrumental music played at a low volume will encourage open, honest conversation. It's nice to have something to listen to when gaps in the conversation occur, but you don't want it to overpower what you're trying to achieve... connection, joy, and peace.

## Make Music

In our workshops and seminars, we often speak with people who express a desire to play a musical instrument. Nine times out of ten they add, "But I've just never had the time."

"Why?" we ask.

The biggest reasons most people give are their careers and family. We certainly understand that, but surely everyone can take half an hour a day. Most people in America spend well in excess of an hour a day in front of the television. Why not use a small portion of that time to play an instrument?

It doesn't have to be fancy. A simple keyboard is fine. A guitar. A harmonica. A Native American flute or drum. They're all easy to play, they're inexpensive, and they give you an avenue of expression. Many of you probably have an instrument collecting dust in the attic or garage. You stopped playing it when you grew up. Well, now's the time to dust it off, get it tuned, buy new strings, and play again. It doesn't matter if you've forgotten most of what you knew. It doesn't matter if you ever take a lesson.

Many people tell us, "Oh, I love music, but I'm not the least bit musical." They've been told they can't carry a tune in a bucket or have a tin ear. Nonsense. Everyone is musical. Everyone has a song to sing. And too bad if the music you're making isn't to anyone else's liking. It's for *you*. Don't let anyone discourage you if it's music you yearn to make. Richard was told by a high school music teacher that he had absolutely no talent or musical ability and should give up the guitar. How wrong that teacher was!

You can make music. It's in you. And there is nothing, we repeat, nothing, better for making you physically, emotionally, and spiritually healthy than making music. It can be with an instrument or with your voice. It doesn't matter.

And what better activity to spend time as a family? Making music is a creative, fun, active pastime. Small children love to make music. Encourage it, and play with them. Get some little drums, or a musicmaker (a little harp-like instrument). In the final chapter of this book, we've listed places you can get inexpensive instruments.

Or maybe you want to dance. Don't worry about form or style or anything else. Turn on the stereo, and dance. Let the beat move your feet. Besides being great exercise, dancing makes you happy. It makes you forget your troubles for awhile, and lets you be a kid again.

*Music will transport you
to the heavenly realms,
where fleets of angels
wait to welcome you,
embrace you,
and grant you peace
and healing.*

D. Joseph

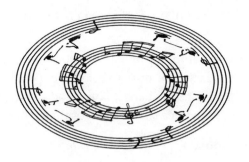

# TEN

# Find Your Healing Sounds

*"The closer I listen, the more profound
the Silence becomes"*

*Anonymous*

Y ou've been enjoying music all your life, but now we're going to teach you how to really *hear* it. You're going to hear the sounds of silence, noise, and finally, the sounds of music. Then, you'll learn to *listen* to all of those things. Let's begin.

Gather this book, a CD player, *"Millennium"* or another CD with which you are familiar, and a pair of earplugs or some cotton for your ears. We'll be doing several exercises in this chapter, but you don't have to do them all at one sitting. The best part about this process of truly experiencing music is that it is ongoing. And any time you feel you need or want it—it's there. It will help you tune in to the joy and peace that are within you all the time.

## A Time for Peace

In this world of eighteen-wheel trucks, airplanes and trains, traffic noise, air conditioners, and dishwashers, we sometimes forget what it is to listen to silence. The sad fact is, many people just cannot bear to be in the silence. How many people do you know who say, "I just keep the TV on for company"? We know many people who have the TV on for the pictures, then mute it and play the radio. Audio and visual stimulation. Doesn't leave the mind much room for introspection and reflection, does it?

First, you must turn things off. Distance yourself from the noise, the clatter, the world. Go somewhere quiet, or at least as quiet as you can find. If you have a family, you'll have to establish ahead of time that you need a little time just for you. Dim the lights or light a couple of candles. If you're outside, make sure you have a hat or are sitting in the shade so that the sun isn't shining right into your eyes.

Now, just sit. On the floor, in your favorite chair, resting with your back against a friendly tree. Sit comfortably, and just like your mother used to tell you, sit up straight. It's important when listening to have good posture. Don't cross your legs or curl them up under you. Wear loose, comfortable clothing. Let your arms rest comfortably at your sides. The idea is to not restrict your circulation in any way and to allow your energy to flow freely up and down your body. Listen to the environment for a few moments before you follow the next steps.

## Breathe

When was the last time you took a really deep breath? Unless you practice yoga or are a long distance runner, you probably don't use your full lung capacity. Take a long, deep breath in through your nose, filling your diaphragm completely, so that your stomach is distended with the air. Hold it a couple of seconds, then exhale completely, blowing out through your pursed lips, until all the air is gone. Repeat this about three times. You will most likely feel a little lightheaded if you aren't used to deep breathing. That's all right. It's because you're bringing extra oxygen into your body.

## Relax

Now, relax your body, one area at a time. Tighten up your face and neck muscles. Hold it a couple of seconds, then relax them. Let your jaw slacken, and your muscles relax. Now, tense up your shoulders and upper back, hold it, then relax. Continue on down your body, first tensing, then relaxing your stomach muscles, thighs, calves, feet. Remember to keep breathing as deeply as you can while you're doing this. When you're finished, go back up to the top and yawn, long and deep.

Rub your temples, your cheeks, your outer ears, massage the area in front of and behind your ear opening, gently. Continue breathing deeply, and gently rub the back of your neck and skull. Gently massage the sides of your neck. Visualize as you do this, that the muscles around the openings of your ears are relaxing, the canals are opening, and the passageways are completely clear and clean. Nothing is constricting them. Envision them meeting somewhere in the middle of your head, and that your brain can pick up all of the sounds they are carrying. The idea is to make the muscles that surround your hearing mechanism relax and be open for better reception.

## The Sounds of Silence

Now, just listen to the silence. Sit perfectly still for a few moments, listening to the space you're in. It will sound different than it did when you first sat down. You may hear the singing of birds, a cicada chirping, an air conditioner humming. Whatever. There may be many underlying sounds.

Listen to each of them in turn, focusing on each one, then tuning them out. What we're trying to get you to do with this exercise, is just *be aware* of hearing. Listen to all of the sounds around you. Do not try to judge them as good or bad, just *hear* them.

*"Sure there is music even in the beauty
and the silent note which Cupid strikes,
far sweeter than the sound of an instrument.
For there is music wherever there is harmony,
order, or proportion.
And thus far we may maintain
the music of the spheres.*

Sir Thomas Browne

## Listen to your Body

Now put some cotton or earplugs in your ears. This allows you to focus on the sounds that your body makes while it is resting.

There are rhythms and cadences that you can willfully change. You know you can change your rate of breathing, but what about your heartrate? Can you slow it down? Can you think calming thoughts and make your blood pressure lower? Try it. Imagine yourself in a beautiful glade, being bathed in warm sunlight, a gentle breeze tickling your hair. Pay attention to your heartrate and breathing as you imagine this situation. Is it any different from your normal state?

The goal of this exercise it to make you aware of your own body. It's a marvelous gift, this human body, no matter what its perceived faults or attributes. It has its own natural resonating frequency, and we want you to recognize what that is. If you are tuned into what your body is like at rest, you can better analyze what effect sounds and music have on it when it is not at rest.

Then, you can objectively analyze what's best for it, and what you need to avoid. With that knowledge, you can use other tones and frequencies, and music itself, to guide your mind and body to a peaceful, healthy state.

## Listen to the Music

Next, listen to *"Millennium."* Track ten (*Gabriel's Lullaby*) is particularly good because it is simple, and with pure tone. Allow your ears to adjust to hearing music. Keep the volume low. Experience how different it is to listen to this music this way as opposed to the way we normally hear music, without consciousness. This music listening exercise is especially powerful if you can use thick, padded headphones. They not only block out any extraneous noise, but also allow you to hear each part of the music.

Listen next to a recording you have heard many times before. Maybe a pop album, or classical, or anything else you know well. You'll be hearing many more things in it with this new awareness. How does this music make you feel? What kind of frequencies is it sending to you? Once you've finished this part of the listening exercises, take a break. Allow your mind to remember and appreciate the experience of conscious listening.

> *"You are the music*
> *while the music lasts."*
>
> *T.S. Eliot*

## Make your own Music

You've listened to the sounds of silence, to music, and to your own body just being. You've learned to relax your muscles, and make your ears really hear. Now, you're going to feel the vibrations of music within your body, as you make your own kind of music. Do the breathing, relaxing, hearing, and listening exercises as set out earlier in this chapter.

Instead of listening to recorded music, hum. Anything. The tune to *"Amazing Grace,"* if you want or *"Mary Had a Little Lamb."* A favorite hymn. Notice how it feels in your throat, in your ears, even as it resonates in your skull. Now, plug your ears or hold your hands over them, and hum again.

Raise and lower the pitch on your humming. Hum a single tune in its entirety, or pieces from many different tunes. Since your body has now been conditioned to awareness, you should be able to discern the effects of different frequencies in the humming. Which frequencies make your body feel better; which make it feel worse?

Humming is a very effective way to get in touch with your body and the frequencies it needs. But it is also a great way to mask frequencies it doesn't want. For example, if you're in an especially noisy environment such as a subway, or somewhere with high frequencies that are bothering you, hum. You can hum so quietly as to not bother anyone else, but it will still vibrate in your body, and in your mind. You can counteract the bad vibrations by creating your own good vibrations with your humming.

## Enjoy the Music

Now that you've had a chance to analyze what makes you relaxed, what makes you happy, and what makes you sad, it's time for some fun. It's time to listen to some new music. Go to a music store which allows you to sample the CDs. Analyze carefully how each piece makes you feel.

Go to a cafe or other intimate venue where you can hear live acoustic music. There are many talented musicians out there playing soothing, instrumental music. Have a cup of coffee or tea, and really listen to them play. Save the conversation for their breaks.

If the music makes you feel right, find out if the artists have a CD and take it home. Just because it's not in the record stores, doesn't mean their music isn't inspiring. In the last chapter, we mention a few artists who produce music that promotes healing and inner peace. Start there and experiment with others you find along the way.

The main thing to remember when you're choosing music for physical, emotional, or spiritual healing, is that it is inspirational to *you*. Something that has healing vibrations for one person is not necessarily what *you* need. As you practice conscious listening, you will become very good at recognizing what's best for you.

131

*He who has been initiated into the truth*
*knows that to every ripple of melody,*
*to every billow of harmony,*
*there answers within him,*
*out of the Sea of Death and Birth,*
*some eddying immeasurable of*
*ancient pain and pleasure.*

Paul Elmer More

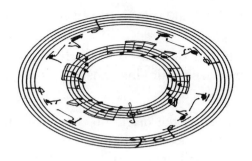

## ELEVEN

# Creating Inner Peace

*"Music is the gateway between your
physical existence and the higher
octaves of your being."*

*Catherine Winkler*

Music is, in and of itself, a powerful healer. Simply by sitting back and enjoying music, you are soothed and comforted.

When you combine the magic of music with the power of meditation and other methods of connecting to the power that is within you, the possibilities for growth and healing are endless.

If you already meditate, you may know most of the material that follows. But if you're new to this whole process, you will enjoy this crash course in consciousness raising. Use this information to magnify the benefits of your musical journey to health and inner peace.

## A Meditation Primer

Don't let the word meditation scare you off. It's not some mystical, secret ritual practiced by a secluded colony of brown-robed monks, as Richard used to think. It's so much simpler than that. Meditating is not "New Age" or complicated or mysterious, and you don't have to fold yourself into a pretzel to practice it.

To meditate is to stop your mind from becoming lost in random thought, and instead, to focus on your consciousness. To go inward and listen is to meditate. By simply being still, breathing deeply and freely, sending conscious thoughts out into the universe, and also allowing them to enter, a magnificent feeling of connection to the universe and oneself is experienced. The gift of meditation is inner peace and spiritual wisdom.

Meditate frequently during the day, whenever you get a few moments to yourself, or in the evening to help relax. Now that he's given it a chance, meditation has helped Richard immensely as a songwriter, dealing with everyday problems, and with matters of the spirit.

There are hundreds of books on the market that teach you how to meditate, but basically there are three methods. When you are beginning this practice of meditation, experiment with all three. One of them will suit you more than the others. Also, one may work for you one day, while another method will work better the next day. The main thing to realize is that your mind will be very, very busy at first. You know, that chatter that goes on in your head when you lie down at night, or when you just sit still. That's to be expected. It will come and go. Meditative, free-form music will help immensely to quiet that chatter. Use the music as you try these techniques.

## Focus on Breathing

Consciously exhale all the air from your lungs. Then, breathe deeply, expanding your diaphragm to inflate your lungs. (Your stomach should be distended here – not your chest!) Hold this energizing air until you feel satiated. Exhale, then, using your diaphragm to push out all of the air from your lungs. Repeat this process four or five times.

Now, just breathe normally, but notice when you exhale. When you breathe out, imagine that all of your struggling—for answers, for success, for anything—is going out. Imagine that the thoughts and emotions that bog you down are being exhaled with your breath. Before you breathe in, there will be a slight gap—an open space—where you stop struggling and surrender. As you breathe in, expand that gap. Expand that open space so that your mind can relax.

Focus only a small part of your attention on the actual breathing. The rest, focus on that gap in thought, where your mind is set free. As you practice this, you will find that the gap gets longer and longer, and your mind is open to the important thoughts that you may wish to focus on. This is where the real meditation comes.

## Focus on an Object

Many of us need to focus our vision on an object in order to clear the mind. A burning candle, crystal, or a piece of art. A painting of an angel, Jesus, Buddha, or anyone else you consider worthy of emulating, or who has brought you comfort and/or knowledge in the past.

Breathe deeply, but instead of focusing on your breath, focus your attention on whatever object you have chosen. As you gaze at it, your mind will initially wander. When it does, bring your attention back to the object. Just as there is a gap between exhaling and inhaling, there is a space between thoughts that come in and out of your mind. That is the free space to which you are aspiring. Expand those free spaces to longer and longer moments of peace. That is where your awareness comes. That is where you meditate.

## Recite a Mantra

In many established religions, including Tibetan Buddhism, Hinduism, and even in orthodox Christianity, mantras are used to focus. A mantra is very simply defined as, "that which protects the mind." It protects the mind from negativity or from the self.

A mantra can be a prayer, an affirmative chant, or even just a few very special words. Have you ever noticed yourself praying fervently, over and over, when you are frightened, nervous, or disoriented?

Kate often says the *Serenity Prayer* when she is frustrated. It makes her feel more peaceful and not so impatient.

*"God grant me the serenity*
*to accept the things I cannot change,*
*the strength to change the things I can,*
*And the wisdom to know the difference."*

The *"Lord's Prayer"* is also a mantra. Many people, especially if they have been raised as Catholic, say a prayer to the Virgin Mary: *"Hail Mary, full of grace, the Lord is with Thee..."*. That, too, is a mantra. Reciting a mantra can completely change your state of mind. It transforms the energy and atmosphere of the mind, because it is the embodiment—in sound—of a truth that you hold. Every word, every syllable, has spiritual power and the mind sends that subtle power to every channel of the body. Chanting a mantra also sends that energy to your mind.

You can recite a mantra slowly and quietly, breathing in and out with the energy it creates. Your awareness, your breath, and the chant will slowly become one. Or, you can chant a mantra in an inspiring way, perhaps even putting it to music, then rest in the silence that follows. That is where your awareness will come.

Some of the most inspiring mantras come from Tibetan Buddhism. Others that we have found to be very powerful are:

*"The Light is me, I am the Light."*

*"Thank you, Great Spirit, for the peace in my soul,*
*the strength in my body, and the joy in my heart."*

You will have other truths that you hold; positive knowledge that you can put into a mantra that will give you strength. Think about them, form them into a mantra, and use them.

## Guided Imagery

Guided imagery is being used in technical ways by many psychiatrists, physicians and music therapists. They help people with specific physical and emotional problems such as fear of flying or arachnophobia. We've created some specific imageries for our own healing work, and included several in earlier chapters, for specific problems.

But the imagery that follows here is a kind of "general use" image. It will take you to a place of peace, and you can use this image any time that you feel a need to get away from things.

## A Journey in Your Mind

As always, before you start, we recommend that you use headphones and play *"Millennium."* Get comfortable, breathe deeply and relax.

*In your mind, you are in your place of work or at home. The normal sounds are all around you, familiar sights and smells. You walk forward, and as you do, the everyday sights and sounds dissolve around you, as you walk into a sea of muted, pastel colors. All around you is soothing, liquid color. You feel like you're walking on a cloud. Weightless, painless. You continue to walk for awhile, and your body relaxes and melds into these soft colors. You are one with your environment, and you are whole.*

*Gradually your body solidifies again, out of the light colors you have just been in. As it does, you see a beautiful green forest before you. You walk out of the muted colors, and into an opening in the forest. You go through the opening in the trees, and follow a comfortable path deeper into the forest. You see friendly woodland creatures around you. They are not afraid of you, and you have no fear of anything in the forest. It is quiet, serene, and has the beautiful scent of pine.*

*You walk further into the forest, and come upon a glade in which there is a small pool. You find a grassy spot beside the water and sit down. You can see yourself in the water, and you see that you are whole, and perfect, and happy. As you gaze into the water, you realize that this place of peace is within you—you have created it. You stand up, smiling, and walk away from the pool. This wonderful, peaceful feeling stays with you, and as you come back to your everyday world, you maintain the knowledge that this place of peace is yours to visit anytime, because it is within.*

Give yourself a couple of moments after completing this imagery before going on with your daily routine. Savor the feeling you have here, and take it with you. If you enjoy this way of meditating, there are many wonderful books and recordings on the market which have marvelous journeys to help you through different challenges in your life.

## Affirmations

An affirmation is a positive thought; a statement of the way things are, or ought to be. Affirmations are often used when one is trying to overcome an illness, an unpleasant state of mind, or a difficult situation.

For example, if you are having trouble learning a new skill at work, or feel in some way unable to accomplish a specific task, a good affirmation would be:

> *"I am a capable, intelligent person. I am ready, willing, and able to perform any task with joy and enthusiasm. I am delighted to have a challenge, and embrace this opportunity to learn."*

It's easy to get caught up in the negativity and unpleasantries that seem to pervade all of modern life. School shootings, natural disasters, gang violence. All of these things work to disrupt our peace of mind. A good idea is to use an affirmation daily to protect yourself from that which threatens to shatter your peace.

Here's an affirmation that Richard uses every day:

> *"I am surrounded by and filled with the pure white Light of the Creator. Nothing but good will come to me, and nothing but good will go from me."*

You will have your own special situations, whether they are emotional or physical. Address them, then put all of the possibilities in a positive light. Put that positive energy into words, and create your own affirmation. We've given you some powerful affirmations in Chapter Twelve, classified by particular problems or circumstances. Feel free to adapt them to suit yourself.

Affirmations may at first glance seem the same as mantras, but they aren't. A mantra is like a chant—something you repeat over and over in kind of a sing-song fashion. An affirmation is a statement.

When you say them out loud, affirmations are especially powerful. Affirmations are always said in the positive. That means, you say, "I am healthy" instead of "I am not sick." Our mind uses the energy from a positive statement much more powerfully than a negative one. As we said, sound is energy. Energy creates. Words create. If you affirm something aloud, then all of the creative energy that is yours flows out from you. The power to create is magnified a thousandfold by your words.

## Contemplations

In the following chapter, we offer some contemplations to incorporate into your daily music and meditation routine. There's nothing magical about them—they are merely quotes, thoughts, and observations upon which you may wish to meditate. They are passages from a book, a newspaper article, a poem, or even off the Internet. Some of them are thoughts which came to us during dreams, or vision quests. We've found that these and other similar passages help us focus when we meditate, and we hope they help you as well.

Searching out your own contemplations is a positive way to spend some time. You'll find personal topics to think about on calendars, in day-timers, in the lyrics to a popular song, or in something your grandmother said when you were ten.

♪ *Perhaps it is*
*music*
*that will save*
*the world.*

*Pablo Casals* ♪

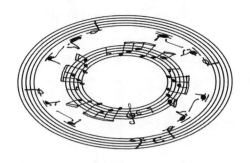

## TWELVE

# The Sound of Healing

*"The work itself is where the joy resides.*
*It is the act of creation,*
*not the creation itself, which gives life meaning.*
*Being at peace is not a goal.*
*It is an ongoing act of creation."*

*Kate Mucci*

This is our favorite part of the book. Here's where you get to put into action all of the wonderful information you've learned so far.

In Chapter Nine you learned how to make your environment more peaceful. Chapter Ten taught you how to hear and listen… and to make music. You've learned to be aware of the effects that sounds have on your body, your mind, and your spirit. In Chapter Eleven you took a crash course in consciousness raising.

Now, with this new awareness and ability to truly listen to music, we are offering to you a series of beautiful inspirations and imageries that you can use while you're listening to music. Use them to take you away from the here and now, to help you connect to your inner self, to reduce stress, and to generally feel more positive and whole.

## Healing and Inner Peace

The following meditations, music, and other tools are offered here to help you on your journey to inner peace and optimum health.

Remember, this journey is a very personal one. Everything we suggest here is very much subject to your own interpretation, and you must adapt it to your specific lifestyle. The most important thing is to take time for yourself, and to know that your quest for health and peace is worth every moment.

Enjoy the recorded music we've recommended. Explore the other artists and genres of music that are available to you in your local stores and through the Internet. Make your own kind of music. Sing. Hum. Bang a drum. Blow on a harmonica. Strum an autoharp.

Music truly is a gift; unwrap it and enjoy!

## ☛ MORNING ♪

**Recommended Music:**

"*Casle of Keys,*"[1] Ed Achrem
"*Harpestry, A Contemporary Collection,*"[2] various artists
"*Celestial Winds I,*"[3] Lisa Franco

**Morning Meditation:**

This isn't so much a meditation as a gentle awakening. Most of us don't have time to get into a focused meditation first thing in the morning. However, if you gently awaken your body, and treat your mind and soul to soft music before tackling the day, you will be much better prepared to face the challenges the day may bring.

For five minutes, before you get out of bed, awaken your body slowly. Focus on each of your body parts, your toes, your legs, your arms, your spine. Flex and relax them one at a time. Shrug your shoulders, squint your eyes, clench and relax your jaws. Then, when you do arise, do so slowly, stretching out your limbs and spine. Warm them up, treat them gently and with gratitude for cooperating.

**Contemplation:**

Instead of listening to or watching the morning news and thinking about all of the terrible things that occurred in the world overnight, or what may happen today, imagine positive, constructive events in your own life and the world.

Time is a relative thing. To appreciate the meaning of a second, talk to someone who has survived an accident. To appreciate the meaning of a year, talk to someone who has just lost the love of their life. Remember that each moment is a precious gift, a breath of happiness.

**Affirmation:**

I am grateful for this day, and for the opportunities it gives me to learn, to grow, and to experience joy. I am healthy, strong, and at peace.

**Mantra:**

Peace and Harmony are mine.

## ♭ AFTERNOON ♪

**Recommended Music:**

*"Matriarch,"*[4] Joanne Shenandoah
*"Wolf Song,"*[5] Nature Quest
*"The Visit,"*[6] Loreena McKennitt

**Contemplation:**

If I make life look easy, it will become so.

**Affirmation:**

Today, now, I release all of my anger, guilt, and fear. I am relaxed and peaceful. I continue my day with Joy.

**Mantra:**

Do unto others that which is the best for everyone.

## ♪ EVENING OR NIGHT ♪

**Recommended Music for simple relaxation, dinner music, visiting, or napping:**

*"Celtic Twilight 3 Lullabies,"*[7] Various

*"Millennium,"*[8] Crosswynd (the CD included with this book)

*"World Blue,"*[9] Neil Jacobs

**Recommended Music for Meditation:**

*"The Fairy Ring,"*[10] Mike Rowland

*"Rain Forest Meditation,"*[11] Daniel Emmanuel (this is an excellent guided meditation)

*"Celestial Love Songs,"*[12] Brain Mind Research

**Contemplation:**

So much good happens every day. Is it by accident? How many coincidences made my life better today?

**Affirmation:**

As I go to sleep tonight, I know that I am blessed by my own strength and love, and the love of my creator. I let all of my thoughts flow freely tonight. As I sleep, I will embrace the creative power of my dreams. I use my own power to heal every part of myself, and to find and enjoy the peace that is within my Self.

**Mantra:**

I'm glad to be me.

## ♪ PEACE OF MIND ♪

**Recommended Music:**

*"Gifts of the Angels,"*[13] Steven Halpern
*"The Weaving,"*[14] Denean
*"Lifescapes Relaxing Harp,"*[15] Judy Dow and Joel Sayles

**Contemplation:**

"A human being is a part of a whole, called by us 'universe,' a part limited in time and space.

He experiences himself, his thoughts and feelings as something separated from the rest... a kind of optical delusion of his consciousness. This delusion is a kind of prison for us, restricting us to our personal desires and to affection for a few persons nearest to us. Our task must be to free ourselves from this prison by widening our circle of compassion to embrace all living creatures and the whole of nature in its beauty."

Albert Einstein

**Affirmation:**

I know that I can do whatever I am called upon to do; that I can handle whatever I must. I am blessed by confidence and peace of mind.

**Mantra:**

An open door welcomes peace.

## ☞ ANTIDOTE TO STRESS ♪

**Recommended Music:**

*"Millennium,"*[8] Crosswynd (the CD included with this book)
*"Celtic Legacy,"*[16] Various
*"Sound Healing"*[17] or *"Ocean Dreams,"*[18] Dean Evenson

**Meditation Exercise:**

Turn on any of the recommended recordings and follow these steps to completely relax.

Lie down, with any constricting clothing, belts, or jewelry loosened or removed. Close your eyes. Starting at the top of your head, tighten every muscle group. Scrunch up your eyes, cheek, and neck muscles. Hold that for a couple of seconds, then release them. Take a deep breath. Do the same with your shoulders, arms, hands, fingers, every part of your body, including your toes. Once your body is relaxed, use guided imagery to take you to a stress-free place. (See the section on guided imagery in Chapter Eleven and also the imageries in Chapter Five).

**Contemplation:**

With each discouragement comes a golden opportunity to try again. With each chance to try again comes a choice. The choice to approach each challenge with love and joy or with fear will affect how I perceive the outcome.

**Affirmation:**

I am a spiritual being having this human experience. Just as a tourist visits an exotic land, I am visiting earth. All of this is transient, and each day is another experience to contemplate; another photo for the album.

**Mantra:**

Amid the noise and haste, I travel in peace.

There is peace in my heart, and comfort in my soul.

## ♭ GRIEF ♪

**Recommended Music:**

*"The Chant,"*[19] Benedictine Monks
*"In Search of Angels,"*[20] Various
*"Sons of Somerled,"*[21] Steve McDonald

**Contemplation:**

To have suffered a great loss is to feel emptiness. It is all right to feel empty, for then there is room to grow.

Grief itself is an operation of the healing system, and I take this opportunity to heal my own self.

A great challenge when you are grieving is to forgive yourself for losing who or whatever you have lost, and to forgive who or whatever has left you. Be sure to go back and use the wonderful forgiveness exercises and imageries we gave you in Chapter Seven whenever you feel the need.

**Affirmation:**

I am grateful that I had the opportunity to know and love _____. I feel that love now, and hold it close to my heart where it gives me peace.

**Mantra:**

To everything there is a season.

## ♪ DEPRESSION ♪

### Recommended Music:

"*Celtic Odyssey,*"[22] Various
"*The Nature of Hope,*"[23] Susan Mazer and Dallas Smith
"*White Stones,*"[24] Secret Garden

### Contemplation:

"The greatest joy of life is in giving, in loving, and in sacrificing. To give, we must have abundance in ourselves. We cannot give what we have not. Therefore, create fullness: good health, good emotions in plenty, good knowledge. Then, give help to all. Give love and sympathy to those who deserve them, give knowledge to all who need it. Give. To give is life. To take is death."

Swami Chinmayananda

Also, use the listening and forgiving practices in Chapter Six.

### Affirmation:

I am content with the gift I have been given—the greatest gift of all, which is life. The best of everything is mine, for I have the love of the Creator.

### Mantra:

Don't worry, be happy!

## ♭ CALMING MUSIC FOR
## YOUNG CHILDREN AND TEENAGERS ♪

**Recommended Music:**

*"The Book of Secrets,"*[25] Loreena McKennitt
*"The Memory of Trees,"*[26] Enya
*"Forest Rain,"*[27] Dean Evenson

**Guided Imagery for young people dealing with stress:**

Imagine yourself in a totally quiet, natural place. A waterfall is splashing in front of you, creating a great plume of mist. The mist gently caresses you, making your hair, face, skin, and clothes wet. It soaks into you, then drips off. When the water drips off, it drips into the stream at your feet. The water is pulling away all your fears, your bad memories, your anger. As it is pulling all of the troublesome emotions out of your body, it is turning dark, and as it flows into the stream, it colors the stream a darker shade of blue. You watch the troubles merge into the stream as it gets wider and wider, heading toward the ocean. Soon, the dark color of your troubles is absorbed into the ocean, unnoticeable in the vastness that is the sea. Your troubles are gone, and you can relax.

Any time you are getting upset, angry, or fearful, use this imagery to help you release your troubles. There's no reason to hold them in and allow them to build up to explosive levels.

**Affirmation:**

I am a good person. I deserve to be calm, collected, and happy, and I choose to be that way.

**Mantra:**

Serenity is mine. I am serenity.

## ♪ REFERENCES FOR THIS CHAPTER ♪

[1] Castle of Keys, Windsong Enterprises, Inc., 1999

[2] Harpestry, A Contemporary Collection, Imaginary Road Records, 1997

[3] Celestial Winds I, Celestial Winds, 1994

[4] Matriarch, Silver Wave Records, Inc., 1996

[5] Wolf Song, NorthWord Press, Inc., 1994

[6] The Visit, Warner Brothers Records, Inc., 1992

[7] Celtic Twilight 3 Lullabies, Hearts O'Space, 1996

[8] Millennium, Two Wolves Music, 1996 *(the CD included with this book)*

[9] Neil Jacobs, Adena Productions, 1994

[10] The Fairy Ring, Antiquity Records, 1982

[11] Rain Forest Meditation, North Star Productions, 1998

[12] Celestial Love Songs, Brain Mind Research, 1995

[13] Gifts of the Angels, Steven Halpern's Inner Peace Music, 1994

[14] The Weaving, Etherean Music, 1993

[15] Lifescapes Relaxing Harp, Compass Productions

[16] Celtic Legacy, Narada Media, 1995

[17] Sound Healing, Soundings of the Planet, 1998

[18] Ocean Dreams, Soundings of the Planet, 1998

[19] The Chant,"Angel Records, 1993

[20] In Search of Angels, Windham Hill Records, 1994

[21] Sons of Somerled," Etherean Music, 1996

[22] Celtic Odyssey, Narada Media, 1993

[23] The Nature of Hope, Healing Healthcare Systems, © 1997

[24] White Stones, PolyGram A/S Norway, 1997

[25] The Book of Secrets, Warner Brothers, 1997

[26] The Memory of Trees, Reprise Records, 1995

[27] Forest Rain, Soundings of the Planet, 1993

# References

There are many wonderful healing musicians and authors we wish to acknowledge. We've recommended their music and we've utilized their books for research and some wonderful quotes. If you would like to learn more about the miracles of music and healing, we encourage you to read, and listen:

## Books

*"Music and Miracles,"* compiled by Don Campbell, Quest Books, 1992.

*"The Mozart Effect,"* Don Campbell, Avon Books, 1997.

*"The Healing Forces of Music,"* Randall McClellan Ph.D., Element, 1991.

*"Music Physician for Times to Come,"* Don Campbell, Quest Books, 1991.

*"The Secret Power of Music,"* David Tame, Destiny Books, 1984.

*"A Harp Full of Stars,"* Joel Andrews, Golden Harp Press, 1989.

*"The Tibetan Book of Living and Dying,"* Sogyal Rinpoche, Harper San Francisco, 1992.

*"Body, Mind, and Music"* Laurie Riley, Laurie Riley Books, 1998.

## Music

We've mentioned many compact discs in this book; most of them are available through your local store or music outlets such as Borders, Barnes & Noble, or Amazon.com. We have also recommended music by the following musicians who are not so well known. Here are ways to find their music:

| | |
|---|---|
| Dean Evenson | Flutes, Harp, Nature<br>P.O. Box 4472<br>Bellingham, WA 98227<br>www.PeaceThroughMusic.com |
| Daniel Emmanuel | Synthesizers, Meditation<br>P.O. Box 8516<br>The Woodlands, TX 77387<br>www.mindwings.com |
| Ed Achrem | Piano<br>512 S. Tonopah, Suite 300<br>Las Vegas, NV 89106<br>www.cdpiano.com |
| Susan Mazer and<br>Dallas Smith | Harp and Woodwinds<br>PO Box 8010<br>Reno, NV 89503<br>www.healinghealth.com |
| Neil Jacobs | 12 String Acoustic Guitar<br>1487 W. Fifth Avenue, PMB 310<br>Columbus, OH 43212<br>www.neiljacobs.com |

# Sources of Musical Instruments

Here we've suggested a few reputable suppliers of folk and acoustic instruments. Between them, they carry every kind of instrument, and you should be able to find something you enjoy, that will help you achieve inner peace, healing, and happiness.

MUSICMAKERS KITS - Ask for Jerry Brown. Jerry knows us well and will be happy to talk with you about an instrument. He specializes in hand made harps, dulcimers, hurdy gurdys, and psalteries. Kate has two special custom-made Musicmaker's 36 string Gothic Harps and they are by far the best sounding lever harps in the world. You can order instruments already made, or you can do it yourself.

> Musicmaker's Kits, Inc.
> P.O. Box 2117
> Stillwater, MN 55082
> (651) 439-9120
> Web site: www.musikit.com

GRAYSON'S TUNETOWN - A quality, family-owned music store with friendliness, knowledge, and 46 years experience. Ask for Ken Grayson. Tell him we sent you. Grayson's is a full line music store with keyboards, guitars, mandolins, violins, autoharps, and a complete line of accessories and sheet music—including music lessons for just about any instrument.

> Grayson's Tunetown
> 2415 Honolulu Avenue
> Montrose, CA 91020
> (818) 249-0993

LARK IN THE MORNING - Mostly mail order, though they do have a few stores around the northwest. Their catalog is amazing! Just about every traditional instrument you can think of. If you're looking for Scottish bagpipes, Uillean pipes, Middle Eastern, or South American instruments, they have it.

> Lark in the Morning
> PO Box 799
> Fort Bragg, CA 95437
> (707) 964-5569
> Web site: www.larkinam.com

ELDERLY INSTRUMENTS - Mail order/music store based in Lansing, Michigan stocking both modern and traditional instruments. Elderly has the lowest prices on new and used Martin guitars in the world, and the most well stocked strings selection in the country. Call them and ask for their free catalog.

> Elderly Instruments
> 1100 N. Washington
> Lansing, MI 48906
> (517) 372-7890
> Web site: www.elderly.com

MELODY'S TRADITIONAL MUSIC & HARP SHOPPE - Retail and mail order music store with beautiful harps and other folk instruments; a great selection of recordings and instructional music books.

> Melody's Traditional Music & Harp Shoppe
> 9410 FM 1960 W Houston
> Tx. 77070
> (800) 893-HARP (4277)
> Web site: www.folkharp.com

# *"Millennium"* by Crosswynd

In this blend of instrumental songs, ancient melodies are enhanced by beautiful original pieces, played acoustically by Kate Mucci on Gothic Harp and Richard Mucci on 12 String Guitar. Light some candles, and listen with love in your heart.

**Songs**
1. *Carolan's Dream* – Traditional
2. *King's Procession* – Richard Mucci, Two Wolves Music, BMI, 1996
3. *Gartan Mother's Lullaby* – Tradtional
4. *Scarboro Faire* – Traditional
5. *Castle Of Dromore* – Traditional
6. *Night Dreams,* Richard Mucci, Two Wolves Music, BMI, 1996
7. *Fair Lady Kate,* Richard Mucci, Two Wolves Music, BMI, 1996
8. *Greensleeves* – Traditional
9. *Lauda St. Magdalena* – Traditional
10. *Gabriel's Lullaby,* Kate Mucci, Two Wolves Music, BMI 1996
11. *Bonny Portmore* – Traditional
12. *Shule Aroon* – Traditional
13. *Aran Boat Song* – Traditional
14. *Pagan Waltz,* Richard Mucci, Two Wolves Music, BMI 1996

(Total playing time approximately 50 minutes.)

*Millennium* was produced by Richard J. Mucci. Mixed and mastered at Son Songs Studios, Las Vegas, NV.

Musical inspiration by Timber and Kayla... our two white wolves and animal soulmates

For this recording Kate played a custom 36 string Musicmakers Gothic Harp and Richard played a Taylor 555 12 string guitar. Special thanks to our dear friend Bill Chenoweth who lent his sensous keyboard skills on selected tracks.

# Contacting the Authors

Richard and Kate Mucci
4616 W. Sahara Ave., PMB 102
Las Vegas, Nevada 89102

E-mail: cwynd@aol.com

Web site: www.crosswynd.com

To order CD's, cassettes, and other books and music by Richard and Kate Mucci, please contact them at the above address.

The Mucc's perform together as the duo Crosswynd. Kate plays the Gothic Harp, and Richard plays twelve string guitar.

In addition to Crosswynd's candlelit magical music concerts, Kate and Richard conduct workshops and seminars on the therapeutic powers of music. Their company also provides stress reducing music conditioning programs for the workplace.

Kate Mucci is now doing Personal Healing Recordings using a secret set of ancient music codes. These ancient codes were re-discovered two hundred years ago by composers like Haydn, Brahms and Ravel, then lost again until recently. These amazing 20–30 minute recordings turn the letters and numbers of your name and birthdate into musical notes, creating a one-of-a-kind recording for personal healing and growth. Please contact Kate directly for details.

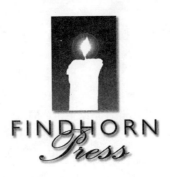

**FINDHORN** *Press*

Findhorn Press is the publishing business of the Findhorn Community which has grown around the Findhorn Foundation in northern Scotland.

For further information about the Findhorn Foundation and the Findhorn Community, please contact:

## Findhorn Foundation
The Visitors Centre
The Park, Findhorn IV36 3TY, Scotland, UK
tel 01309 690311• fax 01309 691301
email reception@findhorn.org
www.findhorn.org

For a complete Findhorn Press catalogue, please contact:

## Findhorn Press

The Park, Findhorn,
Forres IV36 3TY
Scotland, UK
Tel 01309 690582
freephone 0800-389-9395
Fax 01309 690036

P. O. Box 13939
Tallahassee
Florida 32317-3939, USA
Tel (850) 893 2920
toll-free 1-877-390-4425
Fax (850) 893 3442

e-mail info@findhornpress.com
http://www.findhornpress.com